Botulinum Toxin for Urinary Tract Disease: After a Decade from Approval

Botulinum Toxin for Urinary Tract Disease: After a Decade from Approval

Guest Editor

Heinrich Schulte-Baukloh

MDPI

Basel • Beijing • Wuhan • Barcelona • Belgrade • Novi Sad • Cluj • Manchester

Guest Editor
Heinrich Schulte-Baukloh
Department of Urology
Charité University Hospital
Berlin
Germany

Editorial Office
MDPI AG
Grosspeteranlage 5
4052 Basel, Switzerland

This is a reprint of the Special Issue, published open access by the journal *Toxins* (ISSN 2072-6651), freely accessible at: https://www.mdpi.com/journal/toxins/special_issues/07648BYB32.

For citation purposes, cite each article independently as indicated on the article page online and as indicated below:

Lastname, A.A.; Lastname, B.B. Article Title. *Journal Name* **Year**, *Volume Number*, Page Range.

ISBN 978-3-7258-6338-9 (Hbk)
ISBN 978-3-7258-6339-6 (PDF)
https://doi.org/10.3390/books978-3-7258-6339-6

Contents

About the Editor

Heinrich Schulte-Baukloh

Heinrich Schulte-Baukloh, Ass. Prof. of Urology, Department of Urology, and Urologic Private Practice, Charité—University Hospital Berlin, 10117 Berlin, Germany. Special interest in hyperactive bladder function in neurogenic and non-neurogenic patients, especially with the treatment of botulinum toxin A injections, in which he has experience since the beginning of this therapy in 2000.

toxins

MDPI

Editorial

Assessing the Use of BotulinumtoxinA for Hyperactive Urinary Tract Dysfunction a Decade After Approval

Heinrich Schulte-Baukloh [1,2,3]

1 Department of Urology, Charité—University Hospital, 12203 Berlin, Germany; heinrich.schulte-baukloh@charite.de
2 Urologic Practice Turmstrasse, 10551 Berlin, Germany
3 Department of Urology, University Hospital Brandenburg, 14770 Brandenburg, Germany

Botulinum toxin was approved by the Food and Drug Administration in 2011 for neurogenic bladder and in 2013 for idiopathic overactive bladder (OAB). In this Special Issue, we address the question of where we stand with this therapy a decade later. Has it prevailed and been proven useful? Which techniques have become established, and how were they optimized? Are more practical ways of distribution on the way? What acceptance problems or obstacles to long-term use might exist among patients or doctors? What are the risks? Has the therapy gained a foothold in the outpatient sector?

We are pleased to present you with diverse, largely practical aspects of botulinum toxin-A detrusor injections (BoNT/A-DI).

A review by E. Enemchukwu et al. (1) summarizes interesting aspects of various injection techniques from 43 seminal articles. Ongoing debate exists on whether 20 injections are necessary (as recommended in the AbbVie package insert) or fewer would achieve the same results. Based on this work, evidence suggests that fewer injections (comparing 1–10 vs. 20–40) maintain efficacy while reducing treatment time and the associated discomfort and pain. Various injection sites in the bladder lead to different levels of effectiveness, seemingly higher for detrusor (although this may result in an increased risk of urinary retention) than suburothelial injections. These authors believe that including the trigone is safe and effective without increasing the risk of vesicoureteral reflux. This will likely lead to widespread adoption of co-injection of the trigone as a standard procedure, and maybe 10-15 injections might become standard as well.

K.S. Eilber et al. (2) summarize the practical experience of a panel of experts (each with a high weekly patient throughput of 10–20 BoNT/A-DI), who discussed how and when BoNT/A-DI should be introduced to patients as an option for OAB treatment. They also discussed effective procedures for the day of treatment and follow-up care to ensure a positive treatment experience for patients and improve compliance with this long-term therapy. Important best practices include providing patients with clear advice on available OAB therapies, including BoNT/A-DI, during the initial consultation. A practice setting is preferable to an inpatient hospital setting for performing the procedure. Staff involvement (including scheduling through to follow-up treatment) is essential for a positive patient experience and compliance with this repeated therapy. The panel favored viscous lidocaine bladder instillation (diluted with 5 to 10 mL of normal saline) as an anesthetic. Room for improvement may exist to my opinion. According to the experts, up to 20 injection sites are acceptable, but fewer is preferable. Subsequent treatments should be scheduled in a standardized manner from the outset at six-month intervals, with the option of repeating the treatment earlier (at least 12 weeks) if symptoms recur. I suppose, this rigid six-month interval is likely open to discussion.

A practical discussion is presented in the article by M. Oelke (3): Is much of the BoNT/A possibly lost when injected "non-functionally" through the bladder wall into the perivesical tissue? The bladder wall becomes thinner with increasing filling and has a thickness of just 2 mm at a bladder filling of 100 mL—but only in healthy volunteers. Any injection with a longer injection needle of >2 mm and greater bladder filling than 100 mL thus appears to be ineffective into the "periphery". The author's main recommendations are to (1) perform pretreatment ultrasound imaging of the bladder to estimate bladder wall thickness and adjust the injection depth accordingly; (2) fill the bladder as little as possible, ideally below 100 mL(my opinion: makes it difficult to inject the flaccid bladder); (3) use short needles, ideally 2 mm; and (4) provide sufficient anesthesia and pain management to avoid patient movements during the injection therapy.

Time and again, colleagues and researchers have tried to identify predictors of good BoNT/A outcomes to inform patients about the expected success. A wide variety of literature exists on this topic, including men and women. The study presented here by M. Manso et al. (4) presents the results of 368 female patients only. The predictors of efficacy included lower pre-treatment pad usage and the absence of prior sling placement. Repeat injections (at least one) were required by 60.3% of the patients. Thus, only just over half appear to stick with the therapy or repeat it at least once. The average injection interval in this study was 18 months, due to logistical challenges (which raises the question of how patients bridge the interval when the effect of the BoNT/A-DI wears off). Of all patients, 74.5% reported a complete discontinuation of pad usage after treatment, so the rate of 100% continence is outstanding. Importantly, patients who had undergone sling placement were less likely to achieve continence. The low rate of urinary retention (1.1%) and urinary tract infections requiring antibiotics (7.9%) reflects the low-adverse-effect nature of the therapy.

A systematic review and meta-analysis by P.H. Yu et al. (5) of 26 randomized controlled trials and 3,876 patients addresses the adverse effects (especially urinary tract infections [UTIs] and urinary retention) of BoNT/A-DI in neurogenic bladder and OAB patients. The incidence of UTIs in the onabotulinumtoxinA 100 U group of OAB patients was 22.7%, compared with 9.4% in the placebo group (relative risk [RR], 2.53; $p < 0.00001$), with a trend to a higher incidence of UTI with higher BoNT/A doses. The pooled incidence of UTIs in the onabotulinumtoxinA group of neurogenic patients was 48.4% (RR, 1.54), regardless of the dosage used. The optimal regimen of antibiotic prophylaxis within the context of BoNT/A injection seems to require further studies. The most feared adverse effect among patients was urinary retention. Ten studies investigated urinary retention in the context of iOAB. The pooled retention rates were approximately 1.0% in the placebo group, 6.7% in the onabotulinumtoxinA-100U group, and 20.1% in the onabotulinumtoxinA-200U group. The risk of urinary retention was 7.32 times higher in the BoNT/A group than in the placebo group. This is a surprisingly high value, which is unlikely to be reflected in the everyday practice of high-volume centers. Again, the topic of urinary retention thus remains a topic for future research.

Our working group addressed two topics (6 and 7)—the question of pain reduction through the use of thinner needles and the patient-preferred anesthesia method: local versus general. The overall pain score for BoNT/A injections was 2.5 ± 0.3, which is in the very moderate range, and the use of thinner needles could be preferred (assuming otherwise equal quality and practicality criteria). Despite the higher anxiety and pain burden, patients still preferred local over general anesthesia overall.

A completely different use of BoNT/A injections is presented by W.C. Huang et al. (8)—not for the overactive but for the underactive bladder with chronic urinary retention, a condition that we regularly encounter in everyday practice. The treatment of this condition receives too little attention, so this article is worth reading. The authors performed a transvaginal ultrasound-guided external sphincter injection and a simultaneous transurethral bladder neck incision in 16 patients, with good therapeutic results.

Finally, H. Ibrahim et al. (9) present highly interesting and, based on previous knowledge, unexpected results. To investigate the role of SNAP-25 cleavage in the previously known BoNT/A-dependent inhibition of sensory signals, they developed a recombinant form of BoNT/A with an inactive light chain (rBoNT/A (0)), which cannot induce muscle paralysis. They also developed recombinant proteins consisting only of the light chain (LC) domain to better understand the uptake mechanisms, since the heavy chain of the protein is responsible for the internalization of the light chain. They showed that, despite lacking catalytic activity, rBoNT/A (0) inhibited the afferent signaling pathways even more strongly than catalytically active rBoNT/A. This was also evident in the studies of LC-only proteins, where the inactive rLC/A (0) protein inhibited afferent signaling pathways significantly more than the active rLC/A protein. Consequently, immunohistochemistry did not detect cleaved SNAP-25, and purinergic and nitrergic antagonists partially and completely reversed the sensory inhibition, respectively. These data suggest that BoNT/A inhibition of sensory nerve activity in this assay is not due to the classic, well-characterized "dual receptor" mechanism of BoNT/A since it is, at least partially, independent of SNAP25 cleavage and involves previously explored nitrergic and purinergic signaling mechanisms.

We hope that this Special Issue will provide you with an interesting and up-to-date compilation of important topics in urological BoNT/A therapy.

Funding: This research received no external funding.

Conflicts of Interest: HSB is an consultant for AbbVie and regularly conducts workshops for the BoNT/-DI.

List of Contributions:

1. Enemchukwu, E.; Mohamud, H.; Sinclair, S.; Harbour, V.; Syan, R.; Kennelly, M.; Gunamany, S. Intravesical Onabotulinum Toxin AInjection Paradigms for Idiopathic Overactive Bladder: A Scoping Review of Clinical Outcomes, Techniques, and Implications for Practice and Future Research. *Toxins* **2025**, *17*, 211. https://doi.org/10.3390/toxins17050211.
2. Eilber, K.S.; Brucker, B.M.; Pezzella, A.; Lucente, V.; Benson, K.; Kennelly, M.J. Expert Opinions on Best Practices for Overactive Bladder Management with onabotulinumtoxinA. *Toxins* **2025**, *17*, 207. https://doi.org/10.3390/toxins17040207.
3. Oelke, M. Strategies for Safe Transurethral Injections of Botulinum Toxin into the Bladder Wall. *Toxins* **2024**, *16*, 299. https://doi.org/10.3390/toxins16070299.
4. Manso, M.; Soares, J.D.; Henriques, M.; Botelho, F.; Silva, C.; Cruz, F. Efficacy, Satisfaction, and Compliance: Insights from 15 Years of Botulinum Toxin Use for Female Urgency Urinary Incontinence. *Toxins* **2024**, *16*, 332. https://doi.org/10.3390/toxins16080332.
5. Yu, P.-H.; Wang, C.-C. Adverse Effects of Intravesical OnabotulinumtoxinA Injection in Patients with Idiopathic Overactive Bladder or Neurogenic Detrusor Overactivity: A Systematic Review and Meta-Analysis of Randomized Controlled Studies. *Toxins* **2024**, *16*, 343. https://doi.org/10.3390/toxins16080343.
6. Schulte-Baukloh, H.; Weiss, C.; Schlomm, T.; Weinberger, S.; Borgmann, H.; Hoppner, D.; Haberecht, K.; Neymeyer, J. Assessing the Use of BotulinumtoxinA for Hyperactive Urinary Tract Dysfunction a Decade after Approval: A Single-Blind Study to Evaluate the Reduction in Pain in OnabotulinumtoxinA Detrusor Injection Using Different Injection Needles. *Toxins* **2024**, *16*, 395. https://doi.org/10.3390/toxins16090395.
7. Schulte-Baukloh, H.; Apostolidis, A.;Weiss, C.; Schlomm, T.; Weinberger, S.; Hoppner, D.; Haberecht, K.; Waskow, C.; Borgmann, H.; Neymeyer, J.; et al. Assessing the Use of BotulinumtoxinA for Hyperactive Urinary Tract Dysfunction a Decade After Approval: General Versus Local Anesthesia for BotulinumtoxinA Detrusor Injection. *Toxins* **2024**, *16*, 462. https://doi.org/10.3390/toxins16110462.

8. Huang, W.-C.; Tsai, C.-Y.; Chou, E.C.-L. An Alternative Approach for Treating Female Underactive Bladders with Chronic Urine Retention: A Pilot Study on Combined Transvaginal Ultrasound- Guided Botulinum Toxin A External Sphincter Injection and Transurethral Incision of the Bladder Neck. *Toxins* **2024**, *16*, 441. https://doi.org/10.3390/toxins16100441.
9. Ibrahim, H.; Retailleau, K.; Hornby, F.; Maignel, J.; Beard, M.; Daly, D.M. A Novel Catalytically Inactive Construct of Botulinum Neurotoxin A (BoNT/A) Directly Inhibits Visceral Sensory Signalling. *Toxins* **2024**, *16*, 30. https://doi.org/10.3390/toxins16010030.

toxins MDPI

Article

A Novel Catalytically Inactive Construct of Botulinum Neurotoxin A (BoNT/A) Directly Inhibits Visceral Sensory Signalling

Hodan Ibrahim [1,2], Kevin Retailleau [3], Fraser Hornby [2], Jacquie Maignel [3], Matthew Beard [2] and Donna Marie Daly [1,*]

[1] School of Pharmacy and Biomedical Sciences, University of Central Lancashire, Preston Campus, Preston PR1 2HE, UK
[2] Ipsen, Abingdon OX14 4RY, UK; fraser.hornby@ipsen.com (F.H.); matthew.beard@ipsen.com (M.B.)
[3] Ipsen, 5 av Canada, 91940 Les Ulis, France; kevin.retailleau@ipsen.com (K.R.); jacquie.maignel@ipsen.com (J.M.)
* Correspondence: ddaly3@uclan.ac.uk

Abstract: Botulinum neurotoxin A (BoNT/A) is a potent neurotoxin that silences cholinergic neurotransmission through the cleavage of the synaptic protein SNAP-25. Previous studies have shown that, in addition to its paralytic effects, BoNT/A can inhibit sensory nerve activity. The aim of this study was to identify how BoNT/A inhibits afferent signalling from the bladder. To investigate the role of SNAP-25 cleavage in the previously reported BoNT/A-dependent inhibition of sensory signalling, we developed a recombinant form of BoNT/A with an inactive light chain, rBoNT/A (0), unable to paralyse muscle. We also developed recombinant light chain (LC)-domain-only proteins to better understand the entry mechanisms, as the heavy chain (HC) of the protein is responsible for the internalisation of the light chain. We found that, despite a lack of catalytic activity, rBoNT/A (0) potently inhibited the afferent responses to bladder distension to a greater degree than catalytically active rBoNT/A. This was also clear from the testing of the LC-only proteins, as the inactive rLC/A (0) protein inhibited afferent responses significantly more than the active rLC/A protein. Immunohistochemistry for cleaved SNAP-25 was negative, and purinergic and nitrergic antagonists partially and totally reversed the sensory inhibition, respectively. These data suggest that the BoNT/A inhibition of sensory nerve activity in this assay is not due to the classical well-characterised 'double-receptor' mechanism of BoNT/A, is independent of SNAP25 cleavage and involves nitrergic and purinergic signalling mechanisms.

Keywords: botulinum toxin; sensory; bladder; nerve; mechanosensitivity

Key Contribution: This study suggests that the ability of BoNT/A to inhibit sensory nerves is not dependent on SNARE cleavage but rather related to some other activity of the light chain region of the molecule. This unexpected discovery may have important implications regarding the efficacy and potency of BoNT/A when used clinically for conditions in which sensory inhibition may be beneficial (i.e., pain and/or hypersensitivity).

1. Introduction

Botulinum neurotoxin serotype A (BoNT/A) is a member of a family of potent neurotoxins produced by the bacteria Clostridium botulinum (see [1] for review). These neurotoxins are the cause of botulism, a potentially lethal disease resulting in muscle paralysis and asphyxiation [2]. The BoNT/A protein is composed of a heavy chain (HC) of 100 kDa and a light chain (LC) of 50 kDa, each with functionally distinct properties. The HC contains two functional domains, a receptor-targeting domain and a translocation domain. The receptor-targeting domain preferentially targets cholinergic neurons, and, once bound, the translocation domain translocates the LC into the cytoplasm. The paralytic effect of BoNT/A has been well documented and is primarily due to the ability of the LC to bind to and cleave the intracellular SNAP-25 protein, a crucial member of the soluble N-ethylmaleimide-sensitive fusion protein (NSF) attachment protein receptor (SNARE) complex that mediates neurotransmitter release. This leads to the inhibition of the release of acetylcholine (ACh) at the neuromuscular junction, resulting in sustained muscle paralysis. Despite its prominence as a potent toxin, BoNT/A has been used widely in the clinic for cosmetic and medical indications, where its paralytic effects are exploited to provide targeted inhibition of muscle contraction [3,4].

In recent years, BoNT/A formulations have been approved as a treatment for overactive bladder syndrome (OABS), a condition characterised by the symptoms of urinary urgency with or without incontinence and frequent urination. BoNT/A was initially believed to provide relief for OABS by inhibiting the contractility of the bladder smooth muscle via an effect at the presynaptic/parasympathetic level. However, the diagnostic criteria for OABS are largely dependent on the presence of urinary urgency [5], a symptom that is believed to be caused by the hyperactivity of peripheral afferent pathways or by central sensitisation leading to a heightened perception of peripheral input to the brain, rather than muscle contraction [6].

Clinical studies investigating the efficacy of BoNT/A in the treatment of OABS have shown significant reductions in the incidence of urgency [7–11], indicating that, in the lower urinary tract (and potentially elsewhere), BoNT/A may work via a non-classical mechanism, which might not involve the perturbation of ACh release. An experimental study using mouse tissue has shown that BoNT/A can directly inhibit the sensory responses of intramural afferent nerves from the mouse bladder [12]. Antinociceptive effects unrelated to muscle paralysis have also been reported in the literature, where BoNT/A treatment caused a significant reduction in formalin- or carrageenan-evoked pain responses of the rat [13,14].This has been further confirmed by experimental findings that show a significant inhibition of trigeminal neurons following BoNT/A treatment [15,16]. While the effect of BoNT/A on muscle contractility is well documented and understood, evidence from these studies points to a direct sensory effect of BoNT/A that is not sufficiently explained by the inhibition of ACh release at neuromuscular junctions.

The aim of this study was to understand the mechanisms involved in the BoNT/A-mediated modulation of sensory signalling. For the first time, we show that the significant inhibition of afferent nerve signalling was achieved without evidence of cleaved SNAP-25 and by molecules that did not include the receptor binding or translocation domains of BoNT/A. These findings propose a novel mechanism by which BoNT/A may inhibit visceral hypersensitivity without causing muscle paralysis.

2. Results

2.1. AboBoNT-A Directly Inhibited Sensory Nerve Firing from the Bladder

To investigate the effect of 100 U/mL aboBoNT-A on the ability of intramural afferent nerves to detect physiological and nociceptive levels of bladder distension, we used a well-characterised ex vivo preparation that facilitated the concomitant recording of intravesical pressure and afferent nerve firing. The distension of the bladder to 50 mmHg caused a graded increase in afferent nerve discharge consistent with the recruitment of a number of mechanosensitive pelvic and hypogastric afferent nerve units. This typical afferent response was significantly blunted following treatment with 100 U/mL aboBoNT-A. Figure 1A shows a reduction in the mechanosensitive responses to filling 90 min after treatment with 100 U/mL aboBoNT-A. AboBoNT-A significantly reduced mechanosensitive afferent firing over the 90 min protocol (Figure 1B). To explore whether there was a temporal element in the aboBoNT-A-induced inhibition, the levels of inhibition at the measured time points were compared. It was found that, 30 min after treatment, peak nerve firing at 50 mmHg was reduced by 18.2% (±6.23%), while by 90 min post-treatment, nerve firing was reduced by 32.5% (±10.7%). However, the data showed no difference between the action of aboBoNT-A on units firing at physiological pressure (15 mmHg) and at nociceptive pressure (50 mmHg) (Figure 1C). Bladder compliance appeared to be slightly increased following aboBoNT-A treatment (Figure 1D).

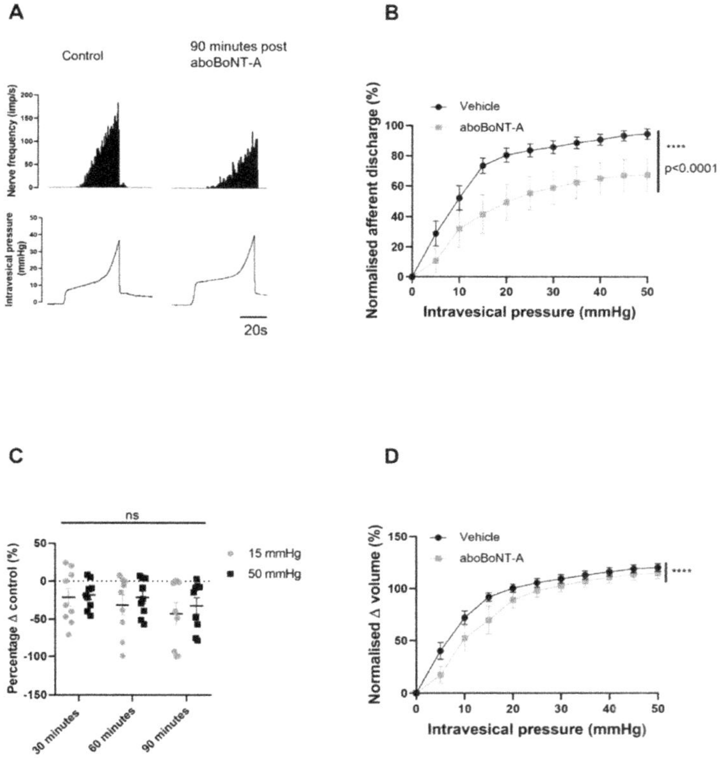

Figure 1. aboBoNT-A directly inhibited mechanosensitive firing. (**A**) A representative trace showing the response of afferent nerves to distension prior to (control) and 90 min after application of 100 U/mL aboBoNT-A. (**B**) Afferent responses to distension were significantly reduced in preparations that received intravesical aboBoNT-A (n = 9) compared to vehicle-treated (n = 13) preparations ($p < 0.0001$; two-way ANOVA). (**C**) Percentage change in peak firing at 15 and 50 mmHg showed no difference between the early and later time points ($p = 0.1003$; n = 9; two-way ANOVA). (**D**) The pressure–volume relationship was significantly lower in preparations that received intravesical aboBoNT-A (n = 9) than in vehicle-treated (n = 13) preparations (**** = $p < 0.0001$; two-way ANOVA).

2.2. Investigation of the Presence of SNAP-25 and cSNAP-25 within the Bladder Wall

Using immunohistochemistry, the expression of SNAP-25 and the cleaved form of SNAP-25 (cSNAP-25) that remains following BoNT/A cleavage was investigated.

As shown in Figure 2, SNAP25 immunoreactivity (SNAP-25-IR) was found throughout the detrusor smooth muscle layers of the bladder wall in a staining pattern reminiscent of nerve fibres. The level of staining was similar between the vehicle-treated control preparations and the aboBoNT-A-treated preparations, which suggests that aboBoNT-A did not affect the expression of the full-length SNAP-25 protein.

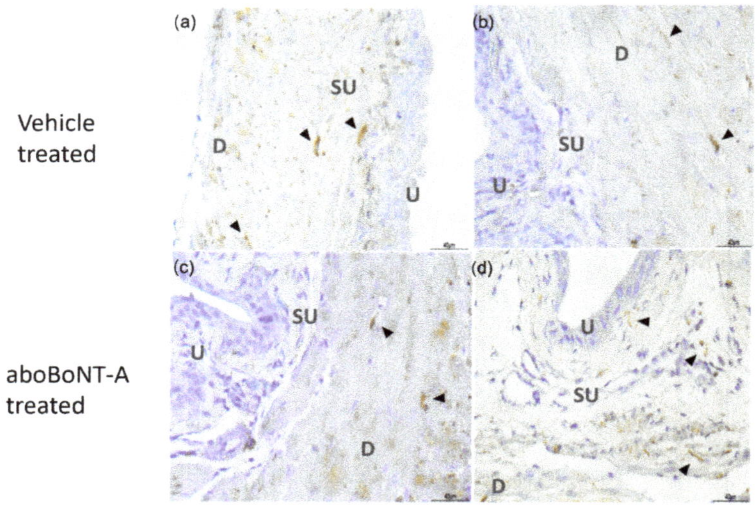

Figure 2. SNAP-25 immunoreactivity in the bladder wall. A representative figure showing vehicle-treated (**a**,**b**) and aboBoNT-A-treated (**c**,**d**) bladder samples labelled with anti-SNAP-25 antibody. SNAP-25 immunoreactivity is labelled by black arrowheads, found predominantly in the suburothelial and detrusor layers. Images labelled as U—urothelium, SU—suburothelium and D—detrusor smooth muscle.

There was no detectable cSNAP25 immunoreactivity in either the aboBoNT-A-treated or vehicle-treated control bladder tissue (Figure 3). The cSNAP-25 antibody was validated as being able to detect cleaved SNAP25 in tissue sections, against sections of rat skeletal muscle from animals previously treated with the aboBoNT-A toxin (see Supplementary Figure S1).

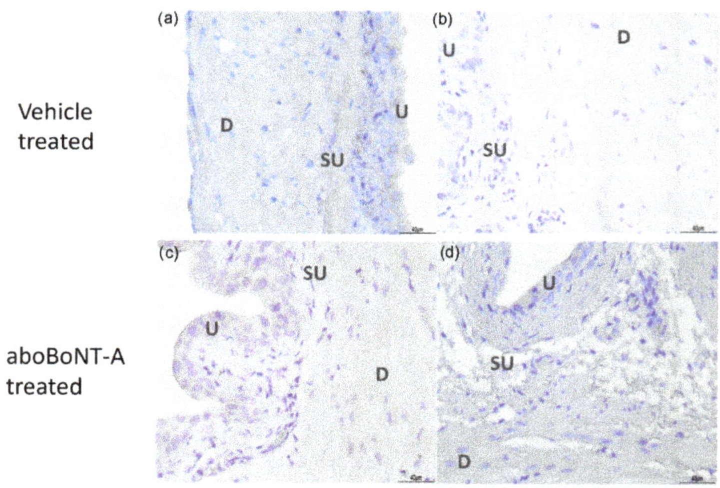

Figure 3. cSNAP-25 immunoreactivity within the bladder wall. A representative figure showing vehicle-treated (**a**,**b**) and aboBoNT-A-treated (**c**,**d**) bladder samples labelled with anti-cSNAP-25 antibody. No positive staining was found in vehicle- or aboBoNT-A-treated samples. Images labelled as U—urothelium, SU—suburothelium and D—detrusor smooth muscle.

2.3. Catalytically Inactive BoNT/A Significantly Inhibited Sensory Nerve Firing from the Bladder

To further investigate whether SNAP-25 cleavage was necessary for the BoNT/A effect on bladder sensory nerves, recombinant catalytically active (rBoNT/A) and catalytically (rBoNT/A(0)) forms of the toxin were generated; rBoNT/A(0) contains the point mutations E224Q and H227Y, which disrupt the coordination of the active site zinc ion and abolish measurable endopeptidase activity [17,18]. We first tested the recombinant toxins on mouse skeletal muscle contractility, using the well-established phrenic nerve hemidiaphragm assay. After incubation with the catalytically active rBoNT/A, the contraction amplitude of the diaphragm was completely inhibited, with a t50 of 24.1 (+/− 0.1) minutes consistent with a cholinergic blockade of the neuromuscular junction caused by SNAP25 cleavage, which has been well documented. In contrast, the application of the catalytically inactive construct rBoNT/A (0) had no effect on skeletal muscle contractility, as there was no difference in contraction amplitude to the buffer control, which was similar to preincubation contraction (Figure 4).

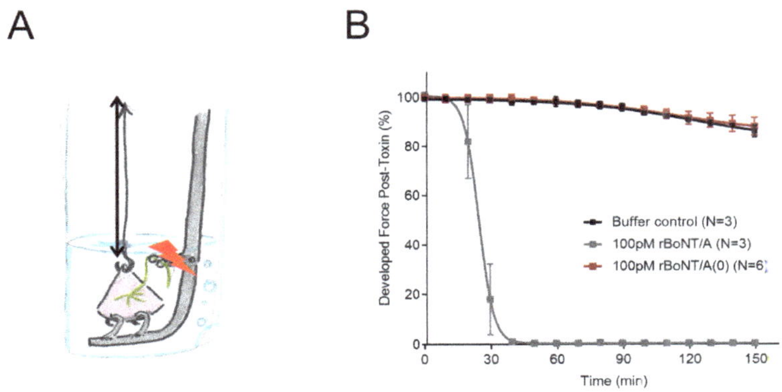

Figure 4. The mouse phrenic nerve hemidiaphragm assay characterising the effects of rBoNT/A and rBoNT/A (0). (**A**) A schematic diagram showing the experimental setup of the preparation. (**B**) The effects of rBoNT/A (n = 3) and rBoNT/A (0) (n = 6) on hemidiaphragm contractility. rBoNT/A1 significantly and completely blocked the developed force after 20 min, which did not recover ($p < 0.0001$ 2-way ANOVA).

Preincubation developed force was inhibited by 99.45% (+/−0.06%) by rBoNT/A1. After three hours of incubation, there was no difference between the effect of rBoNT/A (0) and the buffer control (n = 3) on contraction.

The recombinant toxins were then tested in a bladder assay. The representative traces in Figure 5A,B show that, in the extracellular afferent nerve recordings, rBoNT/A produced a moderate inhibition of nerve firing, similar to that achieved by aboBoNT-A (Figure 1A). This was reflected in the analysis, which showed that 71.5% (+/−9.8%) of afferent firing remained 90 min after treatment with rBoNT/A; this was significant compared to the vehicle-treated preparations (Figure 5C). Remarkably, however, the catalytically inactive rBoNT/A (0) construct induced a profound reduction in the mechanosensitive afferent responses to distension, with 26.02% (+/−5.72%) of the afferent response remaining 90 min after treatment (Figure 5B,C). Rather than showing an attenuated effect (as might be reasonably expected due to the inability of rBoNT/A (0) to cleave SNAP-25), rBoNT/A (0) inhibited sensory responses more potently than its catalytically active counterpart rBoNT/A (Figure 5C).

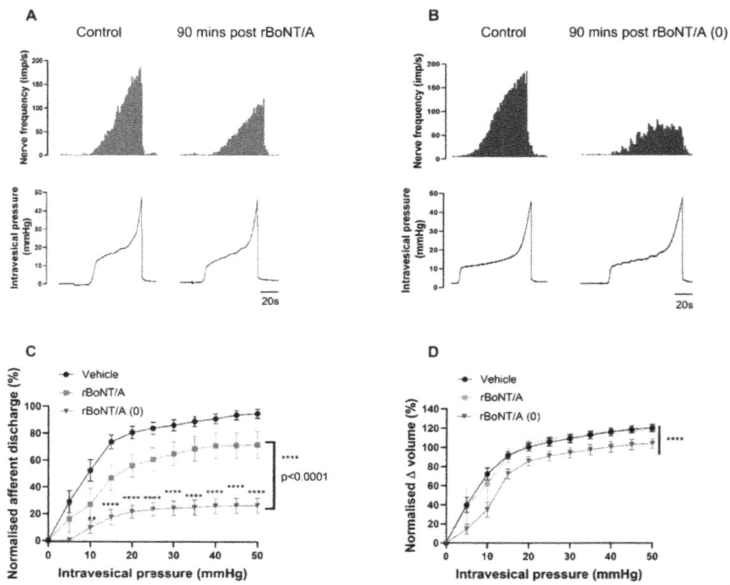

Figure 5. The effects of recombinant active rBoNT/A and inactive rBoNT/A (0) on distension-induced afferent signalling. (**A**) A representative trace showing the response of afferent nerves to distension prior to (control) and 90 min after rBoNT/A treatment. (**B**) A representative trace showing the response of afferent nerves to distension prior to (control) and 90 min after rBoNT/A (0) treatment. (**C**) Distension-induced afferent responses were significantly reduced by rBoNT/A (**** $p < 0.0001$; n = 6; two-way ANOVA) and rBoNT/A (0) (**** $p < 0.0001$; n = 8; two-way ANOVA) compared to vehicle-treated preparations (n = 13). The distension-induced firing in preparations treated with rBoNT/A (0) was significantly lower than in those treated with rBoNT/A (**** $p < 0.0001$) (** $p < 0.01$). (**D**) The pressure–volume relationship of rBoNT/A-treated preparations was not different to that of vehicle-treated preparations ($p = 0.8765$; n = 6; two-way ANOVA), while rBoNT/A (0) significantly reduced the pressure–volume relationship (**** $p < 0.0001$; n = 8; two-way ANOVA).

While the rBoNT/A-treated preparations did not affect the compliance of the bladder compared to the vehicle-treated preparations, rBoNT/A (0) caused a small but significant reduction in bladder compliance (Figure 5D).

2.4. The Light Chains of rBoNT/A and rBoNT/A(0) Alone Inhibited Sensory Signalling from the Bladder

Following the finding that mechanosensory signalling was significantly reduced without the cleavage of SNAP-25, we further explored the role of the structure of the BoNT/A molecule by testing the light chain alone. The catalytically active (Figure 6A) and inactive (Figure 6B) LC proteins inhibited distension-induced firing 90 min after treatment. Like the full-length proteins characterised in Figure 6, the rLC/A (0) protein inhibited afferent firing significantly more potently than the rLC/A protein (Figure 6C). There appeared to be a differential effect on the pressure–volume relationship, as rLC/A (0) was not different to the vehicle-treated preparations, while rLC/A significantly reduced the pressure–volume relationship (Figure 6D). These findings suggest that the receptor binding and translocation domains of BoNT/A (HC/A) are not necessary for the sensory inhibition produced by BoNT/A, and they suggest that the sensory effect is dependent solely on the light chain of the toxin.

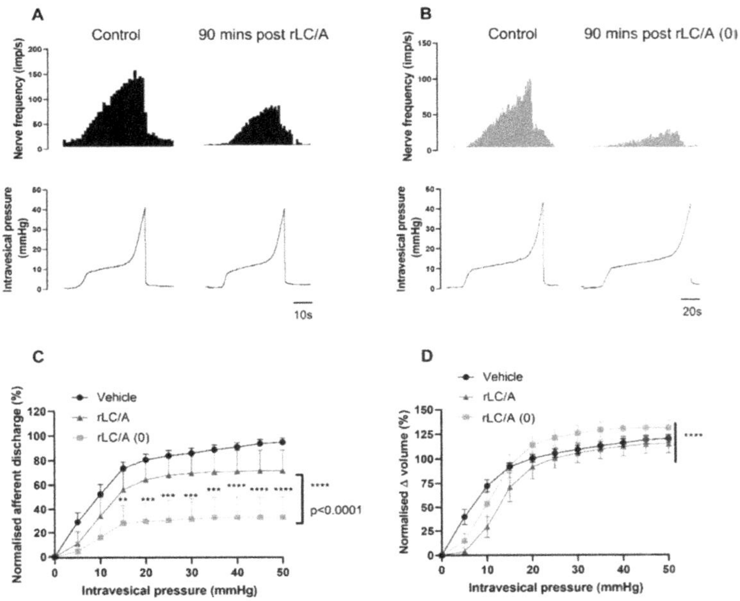

Figure 6. The effect of active (LC/A) and inactive (LC/A (0)) light chains on distension-induced afferent signalling. (**A**) A representative trace showing the response of afferent nerves to distension prior to (control) and 90 min after rLC/A treatment. (**B**) A representative trace showing the response of afferent nerves to distension prior to (control) and 90 min after rLC/A (0) treatment. (**C**) Distension-induced afferent responses were significantly reduced by rLC/A (**** $p < 0.0001$; n = 5; two-way ANOVA) and rLC/A (0) (**** $p < 0.0001$; n = 5; two-way ANOVA). The distension-induced firing in preparations treated with rLC/A (0) was significantly lower than in those treated with rLC/A (**** $p < 0.0001$ two-way ANOVA). (**D**) The pressure–volume relationship of rLC/A-treated preparations was significantly lower than that of vehicle-treated preparations (**** $p < 0.0001$; n = 5; two-way ANOVA), while rLC/A (0) was not significantly different ($p = 0.065$; n = 5; two-way ANOVA) (** $p < 0.01$; *** $p < 0.001$).

To confirm that the observed effect on bladder mechanosensation was due to the activity induced by the light chain domain of BoNT/A, we next investigated the effect of the heavy chain only (HC/A). The application of 3.6pM HC/A did not alter bladder mechanosensitivity (as shown in Figure 7), as after 90 min post-treatment, 89.03% (+/−3.032%) of distension-induced nerve firing remained ($p = 0.9819$; n = 4). The pressure–volume relationship also remained unchanged 90 min after treatment with HC/A ($p = 0.0513$; n = 4). Peak firing at 15 and 50 mmHg did not appear to be altered over time ($p = 0.0927$; n = 4).

2.5. The Inhibitory Effect of rBoNT/A (0) Was Reversed by Nitrergic and Purinergic Antagonists

We applied the non-selective nitric oxide synthase (NOS) inhibitor L-NAME at 1mM prior to and alongside rBoNT/A (0) to assess its effect on bladder mechanosensation (Figure 8A). L-NAME alone did not alter distension-induced firing; however, when applied alongside BoNT/A (0), L-NAME reversed the potent BoNT/A (0) inhibition and led to a slight (ns) increase in mechanosensory nerve firing (Figure 8B). With regard to the pressure–volume relationship, L-NAME alone had no effect (Figure 8C), while co-application with BoNT/A (0) revealed a significant increase in bladder compliance (Figure 8D).

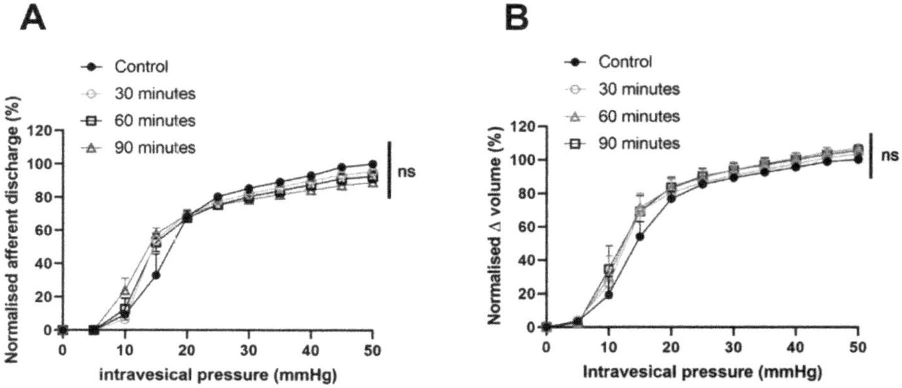

Figure 7. HC/A had no effect on distension-induced firing. (**A**) Afferent responses to distension were unchanged 30, 60 and 90 min after treatment ($p = 0.9819$, n = 4, two-way ANOVA. (**B**) There was no difference in the pressure–volume relationship after intravesical HC/A compared to control ($p = 0.0513$; n = 4; two-way ANOVA).

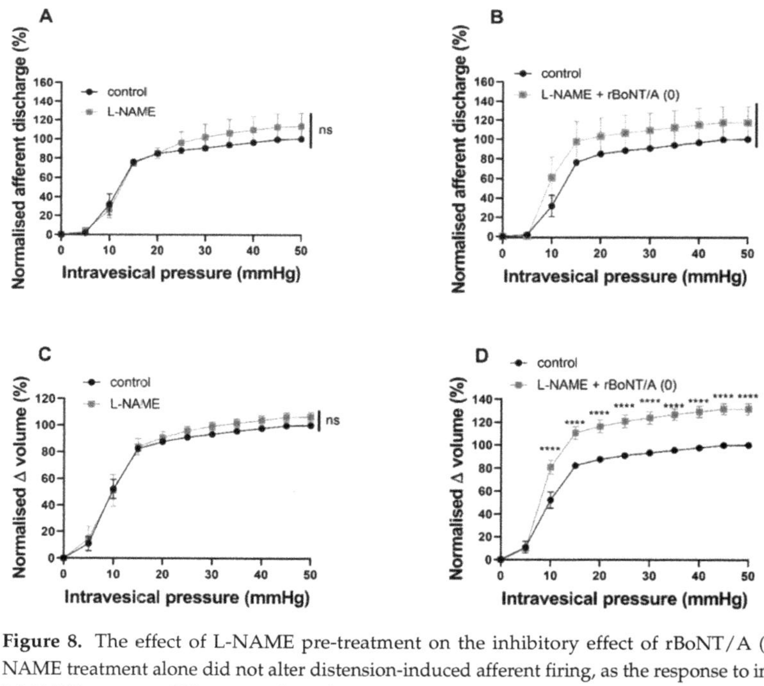

Figure 8. The effect of L-NAME pre-treatment on the inhibitory effect of rBoNT/A (0). (**A**) L-NAME treatment alone did not alter distension-induced afferent firing, as the response to intravesical L-NAME was not different to that of control ($p = 0.475$; n = 5; two-way ANOVA). (**B**) Afferent responses to distension of the bladder following treatment with L-NAME alongside rBoNT/A (0) were not different to the afferent response to controlled distension of the bladder ($p = 0.3881$; n = 5; two-way ANOVA). (**C**) The pressure–volume relationship was not altered by intravesical L-NAME alone ($p = 0.475$; n = 5; two-way ANOVA). (**D**) The pressure–volume relationship was significantly increased following treatment with L-NAME alongside rBoNT/A (0) compared to control responses (**** $p < 0.0001$; n = 5; two-way ANOVA). Sidak's multiple comparisons test revealed significant increases in volume from 10 mmHg (**** $p < 0.0001$) to 50 mmHg (**** $p < 0.0001$).

The P2X receptor antagonist 2′,3′-O-(2,4,6-Trinitrophenyl) adenosine-5′-triphosphate tetra (triethylammonium) salt (TNP-ATP) at 30 μM did not affect distension-induced afferent signalling (Figure 9A) or the pressure–volume relationship (Figure 9C). When TNP-ATP was applied alongside rBoNT/A(0), the potent BoNT/A(0) inhibition was partially dampened. Afferent firing was significantly lower than that of the control but not reduced to the same degree as when reduced by BoNT/A (0) alone (Figure 9B). The pressure–volume relationship was significantly increased by the presence of TNP-ATP alongside BoNT/A (0) (Figure 9D).

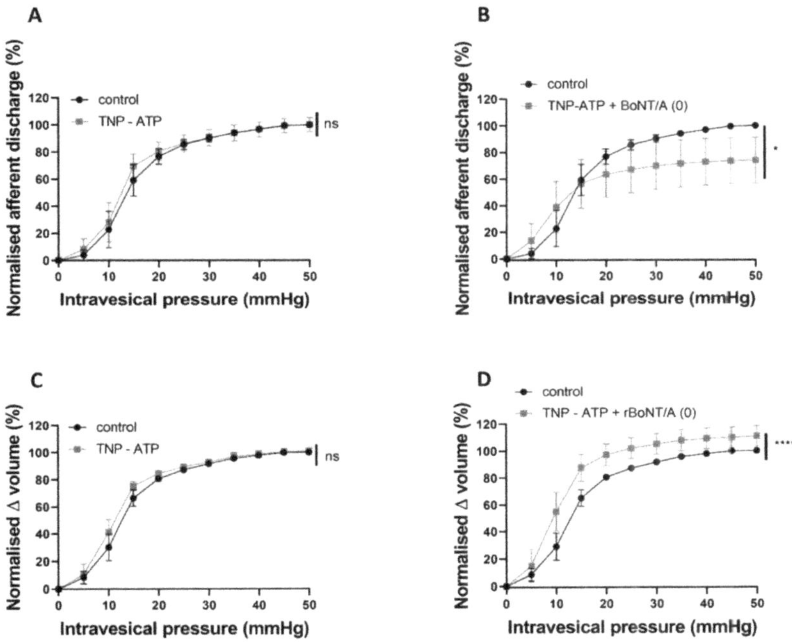

Figure 9. The effect of TNP-ATP pretreatment on the inhibitory effect of rBoNT/A (0). (**A**) The afferent response to intravesical TNP-ATP was not different to that of control (p = 0.4396; n = 6; two-way ANOVA). (**B**) The afferent response to distension following TNP-ATP applied alongside rBoNT/A (0) was significantly lower than that of control (* p = 0.0301; n = 6; two-way ANOVA). (**C**) The pressure–volume relationship was not altered by intravesical TNP-ATP alone (p = 0.2868; n = 6; two-way ANOVA). (**D**) The pressure–volume relationship was significantly increased by TNP-ATP applied alongside rBoNT/A (0) (**** p < 0.0001; n = 6; two-way ANOVA).

3. Discussion

In the present study, we show that a catalytically inactive BoNT/A construct caused a profound inhibition of sensory nerve firing from the bladder. Strikingly, we show that the magnitude of the inhibitory effect was greater than that produced by a catalytically active recombinant BoNT/A toxin (rBoNT/A) or the full BoNT/A complex (i.e., aboBoNT-A). This unexpected discovery may have important implications regarding the clinical efficacy and potency of BoNT/A, particularly in conditions where sensory inhibition is beneficial (i.e., pain and/or hypersensitivity). Moreover, we also show that both the recombinant light chain (rLC/A) and the catalytically inactive recombinant light chain (rLC/A (0)) exhibited the capability to significantly reduce afferent signalling, despite the absence of the typical heavy chain responsible for cell binding and entry. This suggests that the inhibition of sensory nerves by BoNT/A may not be solely dependent on SNAP25 cleavage but may involve other activities within the light chain region of the molecule.

3.1. Abobotulinumtoxin A Directly Inhibited Sensory Nerve Signalling

Abobotulinumtoxin A (aboBoNT-A) is a clinically available formulation of the BoNT/A complex that has been shown to be effective in reducing the incidence of urgency and frequency in clinical studies of OAB patients [9,19];. However, it is not clear whether aboBoNT-A can act directly on afferent nerves innervating the bladder to inhibit mechanosensation, an important component of micturition regulation, the disruption of which is thought to be involved in the development of urgency. In this study, we show that the intravesical instillation of aboBoNT-A into the mouse bladder resulted in a notable decrease in distension-induced afferent firing, consistent with previous findings reported [12]. However, the precise mechanisms underlying the BoNT/A-mediated modulation of bladder sensory signalling remain elusive [12].

As SNAP-25 is the best described target of BoNT/A, we performed immunohistochemistry to look at SNAP-25 immunoreactivity in aboBoNT-A-treated bladders. Our experiments revealed abundant SNAP-25 immunoreactivity throughout the sub-epithelial and intramuscular nerve fibres of the bladder. This is in agreement with previous studies and confirms the presence of SNAP-25 in the mouse bladder [20–22];. Interestingly, however, we found no immunoreactivity for cleaved SNAP-25 (cSNAP-25) in bladders that received the intravesical instillation of aboBoNT-A, despite seeing a clear inhibition of nerve firing; this suggests that either SNAP-25 was not cleaved in these experiments or any cleavage was below the level of detection of this method. The method of aboBoNT-A application might go some way in providing an explanation for this. When aboBoNT-A is used clinically, it is typically injected into the treatment site; however, in this study, we intravesically infused the toxin into the bladder. In a comparative study of BoNT/A application methods, Chuang, (2009), also found that instillation within the bladder did not lead to the immunostaining of cSNAP-25, whereas an injection into the bladder wall did [21]. The lack of cSNAP-25 immunoreactivity within deeper structures within the bladder wall such as the area under the epithelium (known as the suburothelium) and the nerve fibres that lie within the muscle layers following instillation might suggest that aboBoNT-A was restricted to the superficial areas of the bladder wall (i.e., the apical epithelial cells) or that it was working via a non-canonical pathway. It is important to emphasise that these data do not exclude the possibility that SNAP-25 cleavage did occur but that the level was below the limits of detection for our antibody. Further studies are required to irrefutably confirm that aboBoNT-A did not cleave SNAP-25 in this assay using other more sensitive methodologies.

3.2. The Effect of Catalytically Inactive BoNT/A on Bladder Mechanosensitivity

The catalytic activity of BoNTs is dependent on the Zn^{2+} endopeptidase HEXHH motifs within the light chain [23], which have been targeted in previous studies to produce BoNT constructs with little to no catalytic activity [23–25]. Enzymatic activity within the light chain was disrupted through the substitution of essential residues within the HEXHH motif that interact with the Zn^{2+} ion [26]. In the present study, the E224Q/H227Y mutations were made to render the rBoNT/A (0) and rLC/A (0) proteins catalytically inactive [17], which was confirmed using a phrenic nerve hemidiaphragm assay (Figure 4). Contrary to what might be expected, rBoNT/A (0) was significantly more effective at inhibiting afferent firing than active rBoNT/A. This suggests that, when BoNT/A has been rendered catalytically inactive, not only is it able to inhibit sensory nerves, but also the inhibition produced is greater than that for the catalytically active protein. This is particularly surprising given that the only difference between the two compounds was the aforementioned mutation (E224Q/H227Y).

It is possible that rBoNT/A (0) may still be able to enter nerves and disrupt the activity of SNAP-25 despite its inability to cleave it, resulting in a reduced exocytotic release of sensory mediators. However, this does not explain the gulf between the efficacy of the two compounds, especially as the cleavage induced by the active neurotoxin would presumably arrest the function of SNAP-25 more effectively. Previous studies have shown SNAP-25 activity to be unaffected by inactive forms of BoNT/A. Baskaran et al. (2013) found that, while the deactivated recombinant BoNT/A (drBoNT/A) was able to enter motor nerve terminals, it did not affect the release of acetylcholine nor did it inhibit the mouse toe spread reflex [24]. Ravichandran et al. (2015) conducted an in vivo LD50 toxicity assay to characterise their inactive BoNT/A construct (E224A/E262A), finding that it was unable to cleave SNAP-25, as well as being 1.2 million times less toxic than wild-type BoNT/A [27]. These findings suggest that the function of SNAP-25 is unaffected by an inactive form of BoNT/A and that any effects are more likely due to SNAP-25-independent activity.

Although SNAP-25 is BoNT/A's preferential target, it has been shown to cleave murine SNAP-23 at high concentrations in a proteomic cleavage assay and in rat kidney cells [28,29]. In the bladder, Hanna-Mitchell et al. (2015) reported a decrease in SNAP-23 staining post-BoNT/A treatment in rat uroepithelial cells, suggesting the cleavage of SNAP-23 [30]. Thus, one possibility is that, on the apical surface of the bladder, aboBoNT-A targets SNAP-23 rather than SNAP-25, resulting in sensory inhibition. However, the mutation in rBoNT/A (0), which prevents the molecule from cleaving SNAP-25, disrupts the coordination of the catalytic Zn^{2+} ion and removes any proteolytic cleavage ability; thus, it is reasonable to assume that rBoNT/A (0) would therefore also not be able to cleave SNAP-23.

The potent inhibition induced by rBoNT/A (0) was reversed by co-application with purinergic and nitrergic antagonists.

As the rBoNT/A and rBoNT/A (0) compounds are near-identical apart from the substitution of two amino acids, it is reasonable to assume that any effects aside from SNAP-25 cleavage and proteolytic activity may remain in rBoNT/A (0). In the bladder, sensory mediators such as adenosine triphosphate (ATP) and nitric oxide (NO) have been shown to play a role in the modulation of the afferent responses to stretch [31–34]. In the presence of BoNT/A, the release of these mediators has been shown to be altered [12,30,35]. While the release of ATP in the bladder has been shown to occur partly via exocytosis through vesicles and partly through pannexin/connexin hemichannels and other means [36–38], NO release is wholly non-vesicular [34].

By investigating these sensory pathways using purinergic and nitrergic antagonists, we aimed to better understand the SNAP-25-independent actions of rBoNT/A (0). While L-NAME alone did not have any effect on distension-induced afferent firing, when co-applied with rBoNT/A (0), the potent inhibitory effect of BoNT/A(0) was reversed to the point where a slight hypersensitivity to distension was seen. Increased NO release has been shown to be inhibitory to afferent firing [39], while in the present study, L-NAME alone did not affect distension responses. This finding is supported by Yu & De Groat (2013), who found that L-NAME alone did not alter afferent firing in basal conditions but reversed L-arginine-dependent inhibition [40]. It may be possible that rBoNT/A (0) caused NO to be released at a level great enough to potently inhibit afferent firing, which would explain the reversal following L-NAME co-application.

To investigate the purinergic pathway, we tested the P2X antagonist TNP-ATP and its effect on rBoNT/A (0)-dependent afferent inhibition. Again, TNP-ATP alone did not affect distension-induced afferent firing, a finding similar to that reported by Yu & De Groat (2008), who found that both TNP-ATP and PPADS did not influence afferent firing under basal conditions [40]. When co-applied with rBoNT/A (0), TNP-ATP partially reversed the effect, as the afferent firing was significantly lower than the control but not reduced to the extent achieved by rBoNT/A (0) alone. These findings are tentative pharmacological explorations of the potential mechanisms behind the rBoNT/A (0)-dependent effects on sensory signalling, and, while interesting, we recognise that further studies are necessary to confirm these links; however, the data collected do suggest that the sensory inhibition produced by the inactive toxin can be manipulated pharmacologically and may involve the nitrergic and purinergic signalling pathways, raising the possibility that rBoNT/A (0) could also be utilised for the treatment of conditions where nitrergic and/or purinergic signalling is disrupted, including erectile dysfunction (see [41] for a review on use of botulinum toxins as a treatment option for ED), pain and inflammation.

3.3. The Effect of Light Chains of rBoNT/A and rBoNT/A (0) without Cell Binding or Translocation Activities

Another important finding of this study was the inhibitory activity of the BoNT light chains, rLC/A (catalytically active LC) and rLC/A (0) (catalytically inactive LC), on the distension responses of afferent nerves. Both rLC/A and rLC/A (0) inhibited sensory firing from the bladder, but, similar to the full-length proteins, we also found that the rLC/A (0) fragment caused a greater inhibition in nerve firing than the rLC/A fragment. This suggests that the silencing of sensory signalling by BoNT/A involves a mechanism(s) that lies within the light chain of BoNT/A and is not dependent on the full-length molecule.

When used clinically, BoNT/A preparations are normally injected into the site of interest, and the heavy chain of the toxin binds selectively and irreversibly to high-affinity receptors on the presynaptic surface. A 'double-receptor' mechanism has been described [42], where BoNTA initially interacts with glycolipids, such as gangliosides, concentrating the toxin on the presynaptic membrane. Once anchored close to the membrane, the toxin interacts with a second glycolipid and/or protein co-receptor, triggering receptor-mediated endocytosis. For BoNTA, this is the synaptic vesicle protein SV2 (isoforms A, B and C). The necessity of a receptor binding region for cellular entry has been well documented in the literature, with Chaddock et al. (2000) reporting that the removal of the Hc domain in an LHn/A compound led to the loss of internalisation and subsequent reductions in intracellular SNAP-25 cleavage compared to that of LHn/A conjugated to wheat germ agglutinin [43]. However, interestingly, the evidence in the present study reveals that not only is the receptor binding region not necessary, but also the translocation domain is not required to see the inhibition in sensory nerve firing. This finding opens up many potential questions regarding how the rLC/A and rLC/A (0) fragments may have interacted with cells and where they work. It is also unclear how the fragments could have traversed the epithelial barrier of the bladder, which is well recognised as the most impermeable barrier in the mammalian body.

It is possible that distending the bladder beyond a physiological pressure (i.e., to 50 mmHg) causes disruption to the bladder wall, enabling the fragments to reach structures in the sub-epithelial space (i.e., nerve terminals, interstitial cells and blood vessels) or deeper, and that the mechanism of action could be extracellular. For example, the light chain could act as a ligand, binding to a receptor on the surface of a cell to induce a downstream change in NO or ATP release. Over the past few years, interest in novel receptors for the botulinum toxin has grown. Fibroblast growth factor receptor 3 (FGFR3) has previously been identified as another receptor for BoNT/A, with studies showing that a higher FGFR3 expression in neuronal cells can lead to increased toxin internalisation [44]. However, the available evidence to date indicates that it is the heavy chain of BoNT/A that interacts with FGFR rather than the light chain [45]. Moreover, in our current studies, the heavy chain of BoNT/A when applied alone had no significant effect on nerve firing, suggesting that it was not able to either activate a neuronal signalling mechanism or enter a cell.

It is also possible that the LC fragments took advantage of the compensatory endocytosis process, which is initiated during bladder emptying to recover plaques expressed on the surface of the epithelial cell membranes to enter the cells and work intracellularly [46]. However, once internalised, how the LC fragments enter the cytosol or how they exert an effect is unknown.

3.4. Clinical Implications of the Sensory Effects of rBoNT/A (0)

The concept of a non-paralytic BoNT/A that causes the direct inhibition of sensory afferent signalling has significant potential, most importantly in tackling the lack of viable non-addictive treatments for chronic pain. Over the last 20 years, the opioid crisis has spread worldwide, and, often, people struggling with addiction were introduced to opioids following injury or surgery [47]. This illustrates the necessity for the continued development of non-addictive analgesic drugs to stem the growth of opioid dependency in patients, as it is associated with a high risk of overdose and death [48]. The current use of BoNT/A for a host of conditions usually provides long-term therapeutic benefits (i.e., 1–6 months) for patients. While this currently study was limited to a few hours for logistical reasons and, of course, used animal rather than human tissues, if the sensory inhibition identified in this study were to be long-lasting and translatable, then the use of rBoNT/A (0) to treat pain and a host of other hypersensitivity conditions would be a really exciting prospect.

With regard to the treatment of bladder disorders, rBoNT/A (0) offers the potential to provide relief from urgency without the risk of bladder retention, which is an adverse effect reported by patients following an injection of conventional BoNT/A [10]. As there is currently no BoNT/A formulation approved by the FDA for interstitial cystitis/painful bladder syndrome (IC/PBS), further development of rBoNT/A (0) may provide a route to another potential treatment for this indication.

4. Conclusions

This study explored the effect of a novel recombinant BoNT/A construct that has no catalytical activity on the firing of visceral sensory nerves. These data provide evidence indicating that SNAP-25 cleavage activity may not be the driver behind the sensory effects of BoNT/A reported in the literature, as losing that ability did not preclude the rBoNT/A (0) construct from potently inhibiting afferent signalling in this assay. Following continued development and research, rBoNT/A (0) may potentially be used to treat sensory disorders and pain, providing an answer for the lack of non-addictive analgesic drugs currently available for patients.

5. Materials and Methods

5.1. BoNTs

AbobotulinumtoxinA (aboBoNT-A) was provided by Ipsen (Milton Park, UK). Recombinant forms of BoNT/A were produced as described below.

5.2. BoNT/A1 Gene Synthesis

The BoNT/A1 protein sequence (UPI0000001386) underwent reverse translation and optimisation for expression in *E. coli* (DNA 2.0, Menlo Park, CA, USA). The DNA sequence was synthesised in two parts for safety and then combined at a silent KpnI restriction site to form the coding sequence for the full-length neurotoxin. Silent 5′ NdeI and 3′ HindIII sites were incorporated and used to insert the open reading frame into a pJ401 expression plasmid (DNA2.0) to create pJ401-BoNT/A1. The amino acid numbering of the mentioned protein sequences was based on the predicted sequence of the encoded protein, including the initiating methionine.

5.3. Expression and Purification of BoNT/A1

The handling of all materials containing full-length neurotoxins occurred in microbiological safety cabinets situated within restricted-access Containment Level II laboratories. pJ401-BoNT/A1 was transformed into BLR (DE3) cells, expressed as 1L cultures and grown in an animal-component-free culture medium (AF, 12 g/L phytone peptone animal free, 24 g/L yeast extract, 10 g/L glycerol, 76 mM potassium phosphate dibasic and 14 mM potassium phosphate monobasic, 0.2% glucosamine, 30 µg/mL kanamycin) in 2.5 L shake flasks. Expression cultures were inoculated with a 1:100 dilution from an overnight starter culture and incubated at 37 °C with shaking until OD600 0.5–0.6 was reached. The temperature was then lowered to 16 °C, and after equilibrating for 1 h, IPTG (final concentration of 1 mM) was introduced to induce further growth for 20 h.

Cells were harvested via centrifugation (4300× g, 10 min), and cell pellets were stored at −20 °C. The cell pellets were thawed at room temperature and resuspended (3 mL/g) in lysis buffer (35 mM NaCl in 50 mM Tris pH 8.0) supplemented with 10 μL of Benzonase. Cells were lysed via ultrasonication at 4 °C (Misonix 3000 sonicator, 1 cm diameter probe, 10 × 30 s pulses, power setting 4.5, output 60–80 W). The resultant lysate was clarified via centrifugation (4300× g, 1 h, 4 °C), and the supernatant was retained. This supernatant was adjusted to 17.5 mM NaCl, 1.1 M $(NH_4)_2SO_4$ and 50 mM Tris pH 8.0 by adding an equal volume of 2.2 M $(NH_4)_2SO_4$ in 50 mM Tris pH 8.0; centrifuged (4300× g, 60 min, 4 °C); and loaded (4 mL/min flow rate) onto three stacked 5 mL HiTrap™ Butyl HP columns (pre-equilibrated with 1.1 M $(NH_4)_2SO_4$ in 50 mM Tris pH 8.0). The columns were washed with 15 column volumes (CV) of 1.1 M $(NH_4)_2SO_4$ in 50 mM Tris pH 8.0, then eluted over a 20 CV linear gradient (1.1 to 0 M $(NH_4)_2SO_4$ in 50 mM Tris pH 8.0) and collected as 10 mL fractions.

Fractions were monitored by SDS-PAGE (NuPAGE™ 4–12% Bis-Tris gels) stained for total protein (SimplyBlue™ SafeStain, Fisher Scientific UK LTD, Loughborough, UK), and those containing the target protein were pooled and stored at 4 °C overnight. Pooled material was desalted (HiPrep 26/10 Desalting column) into 50 mM Tris pH 8.0 as a series of 11 mL batches. Each batch was collected until the conductivity surpassed 3.0 mS/cm, at which point the column was re-equilibrated until the conductivity dropped back below 3.0 mS/cm for the next batch. This process was repeated until the entire pooled fraction had been buffer-exchanged. The desalted sample was loaded at 5 mL/min onto a 5 mL itrap™ Q HP column (previously washed and charged following the manufacturer's guidelines and pre-equilibrated with 50 mM Tris pH 8.0). The column was washed with 15 CV (50 mM Tris pH 8.0) and eluted at 5 mL/min, 15 CV linear gradient (0 to 300 mM NaCl in 50 mM Tris pH 8.0), and 2.5 mL fractions were collected. Fractions were monitored by SDS-PAGE (NuPAGE™ 4–12% Bis-Tris gels) stained for total protein (SimplyBlue™ SafeStain, Fisher Scientific UK LTD, Loughborough, UK), and those containing the target protein were pooled and stored overnight at 4 °C.

The protein concentration was determined using a Bradford assay, and the sample was concentrated to 9 mL in a Vivaspin 20 centrifugal concentrator (MwCO 5000 Da, 4300× g, 20 min cycles at 4 °C); the protein concentration was measured again using a Bradford assay and adjusted to 0.5 mg/mL with 125 mM NaCl in 50 mM Tris pH 8.0. Endoproteinase Lys-C was added (final Lys-C concentration 0.8 μg/mL), and the sample was incubated for 20 h at 4 °C. The sample was adjusted with an equal volume of 2 M $(NH_4)_2SO_4$ and 50 mM Tris pH 8.0 and loaded onto two stacked 1 mL HiTrap™ Phenyl HP columns at 1.0 mL/min (pre-equilibrated with 1 M $(NH_4)_2SO_4$ in 50 mM Tris pH 8.0).

The column was washed with 10 CV of the same buffer and then eluted over a 15 CV linear gradient (from 1 M to 0 M $(NH_4)_2SO_4$ in 50 mM Tris pH 8.0) at 2 mL/min, and 1 mL fractions were collected. Fractions were monitored by SDS-PAGE (NuPAGE™ 4–12% Bis-Tris gels) stained for total protein (SimplyBlue™ SafeStain, Fisher Scientific, UK, LTD Loughborough UK), and those containing the target protein were pooled, concentrated and diafiltered into phosphate-buffered saline (KH2PO4 1 mM, Na_2HPO_4 3 mM, NaCl 155 mM, pH 7.4) (Vivaspin 20 centrifugal concentrator MwCO 5000 Da, 4300× g, 20 min cycles at 4 °C); the concentration was again determined using a Bradford assay and adjusted to 0.1 mg/mL before storage in aliquots at −80 °C.

5.4. BoNT Constructs Tested in This Study

All of the constructs used in the study were purified using the same protocol as above. For the inactivated toxins, a mutation was made that rendered them inactive in the HEXXH region of the light chain; this involved the substitutions of glutamic acid to glutamine (E224Q) and histidine to tyrosine (H227Y).

Table 1 below outlines the BoNT constructs used in this study. In a series of pilot studies using aboBoNT-A, 100 units/mL was shown to be the dose with the most robust and reproducible response. The concentration of BoNT/A in 100 U/mL was calculated to be 3.6 pM, so this concentration was used in the experiments with other toxins to facilitate comparison ([49]). All BoNTs were dissolved in PBS and applied to the bladders using an infusion pump to fill the bladder to a pressure of 50 mmHg.

Table 1. A diagram describing the composition of all of the BoNT/A constructs used in this study.

Name	Structure	Description	Method of Production
aboBoNT-A	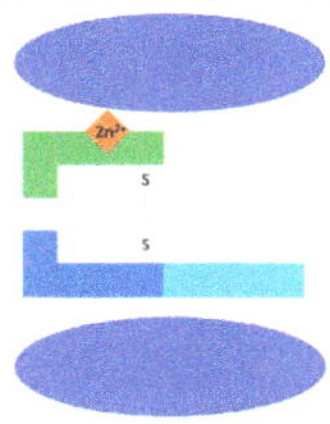	Whole BoNT/A complex, including the non-toxic accessory proteins (NAPs)	Purified from C. botulinum
rBoNT/A	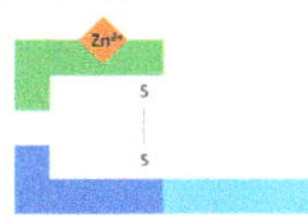	Full-length BoNT/A	Recombinant; expressed in *E. coli* and purified
rLC/A	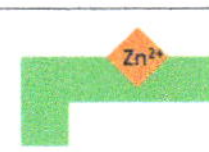	Light chain only	Recombinant; expressed in *E. coli* and purified
rHC/A		Heavy chain only	Recombinant; expressed in *E. coli* and purified
rBoNT/A (0)	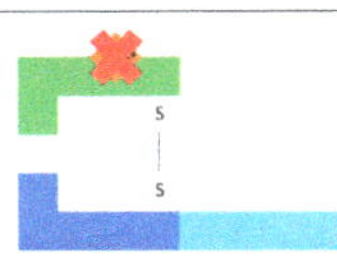	Full-length mutated BoNT/A, catalytically inactive	Recombinant; expressed in *E. coli* and purified
rLC/A (0)	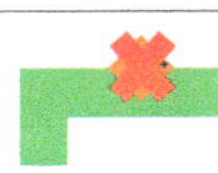	Mutated light chain only, catalytically inactive	Recombinant; expressed in *E. coli* and purified

5.5. Animals

These studies were performed using adult C57BL/6J mice between 8 and 12 weeks old (Jackson Laboratory, obtained from Charles River, Harlow UK). The mice were sacrificed in accordance with Schedule 1 of the Animals (Scientific Procedures) Act UK 1986. Experiments performed were in accordance with the ethical approval obtained from the UCLan Animal Welfare and Ethics Review Board (AWERB) (reference RE/16/11).

5.6. Mouse Phrenic Nerve Hemidiaphragm Preparation

Hemidiaphragm recordings were performed as previously described [50]. Briefly, the left hemidiaphragm and phrenic nerve were dissected and transferred into an organ bath (Emka Technologies, Paris, France). The muscle was connected to a transducer to facilitate the recording of muscle contraction. Electrical stimulation was applied to the phrenic nerve (frequency = 1 Hz; width = 20 µs; 10 V) so as to generate a sustained force of contraction of at least 0.5 g. Following stabilisation and control steps, the sample was incubated with 100 pM recombinant BoNT/A (0) (rBoNT/A (0)), 100 pM recombinant BoNT/A1 (rBoNT/A1) or a buffer control (0.1% BSA in PBS, Sigma-Aldrich, Gillingham, UK) for three hours. Potency is expressed as the time taken to reach half paralysis (t50) using a non-linear regression analysis (GraphPad Prism v8.3). All data are expressed as mean +/− SEM; N corresponds to the number of animals.

5.7. Ex Vivo Mouse Bladder Electrophysiology

Nerve recordings were performed as previously described [12,51–57]. Briefly, the whole pelvic region of the mouse, including the lower vertebrae and urinary tract (kidneys, ureters, bladder, pelvic nerves, urethra), was dissected and placed in an organ bath continually perfused with Krebs solution (NaCl 118.4 mmol/L, $NaHCO_3$ 24.9 mmol/L, $CaCl_2$ 1.9 mmol/L, $MgSO_4$ 1.2 mmol/L, KCl 4.7 mmol/L, KH_2PO_4 1.2 mmol/L, glucose 11.7 mmol/L; obtained from Sigma-Aldrich), gassed with carbogen (95% O_2, 5% CO_2) and kept at ~35 °C. Ureters were tied with suture, and the urethra and the dome of the bladder were catheterised and tied with suture. The urethral catheter was attached to an infusion pump to allow the graded filling of the bladder with phosphate-buffered saline (PBS; Sigma-Aldrich) to 50 mmHg. Ramp distension to a maximal 50 mmHg pressure was chosen, as it has been previously documented to activate both low- and high-threshold afferents, which respond to both innocuous and noxious stimuli [51]. Once that pressure was reached, the tap attached to the dome catheter was opened to allow the evacuation of fluid. The pelvic and hypogastric nerve fibres emerging from the bladder were dissected, cut and inserted into a suction glass electrode connected to a Neurolog headstage and AC amplifier. The signals were amplified and filtered and sent to a spike processor, which discerned signals from noise through a threshold set by the researcher. The spike processor counted the nerve impulses induced by bladder distension.

5.8. Experimental Protocols

The distension protocol followed in the bladder preparations is shown below in Figure 10. At the beginning of each experiment, the bladder was distended three times using PBS to ensure reproducibility, after which the infusion syringe was changed to one containing BoNT solution, and three more distensions were performed. After this, the syringe was replaced with one containing PBS, and distensions continued for 90 min to assess the effect of BoNT on pelvic and hypogastric sensory nerve firing. Any BoNT within the intraluminal fluid was deactivated using Presept (Advanced Sterilization Products) as it came out of the dome catheter.

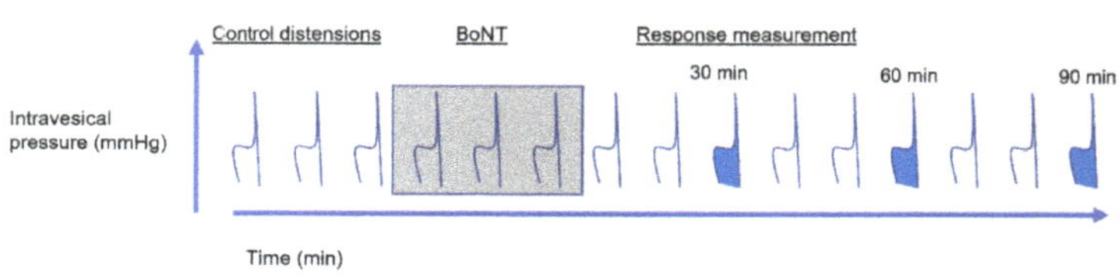

Figure 10. A schematic diagram of the distension protocol. The bladder was distended to 50 mmHg every 10 min throughout the protocol. 'Control' distensions were performed using intravesical PBS; BoNT was applied for three distensions (in PBS, shaded), after which time bladders were then distended again with PBS. The filled distensions in blue correspond to the time points analysed.

5.9. Drugs

N(G)-Nitro-L-arginine methyl ester (L-NAME) and 2′,3′-O-trinitrophenyl ATP (TNP-ATP) were obtained from Tocris (Oxford, UK), diluted in distilled water and stored at −20 °C.

5.10. Data Analysis

The afferent nerve activity recorded from multi-fibre nerve bundles was captured and counted using a Digitimer D130 spike processor, which detected the number of field potentials that crossed a pre-set threshold. Distension responses were analysed using a Spike2 script, and nerve activity at baseline was subtracted from peak firing at 50 mmHg. To analyse the effect of BoNT on distension-induced firing, responses at 30, 60 and 90 minutes post-BoNT treatment were normalised to the control distension before the addition of BoNT. Afferent nerve data are expressed as normalised afferent firing in impulses per second (imps/sec), and bladder compliance was assessed from the pressure–volume relationship during the distension of the bladder. All data are expressed as mean +/− SEM and n number, which refers to the number of animals. A statistical analysis was conducted using GraphPad Prism v.8.0.1, using Student's *t* tests and one-way and two-way ANOVA where appropriate, with a Bonferroni post hoc test. A p value <0.05 was designated to be statistically significant.

5.11. Immunohistochemistry

At the end of the nerve recording, the bladders treated with the vehicle and abobotulinumtoxinA (aboBoNT-A) were fixed at room temperature (~20 °C) in 4% paraformaldehyde (VWR Chemicals, Luton UK) and then kept in 1% PFA/PBS solution at 4 °C. Four aboBoNT-A-treated and four PBS-treated bladders were included in this analysis, dissected from separate mice. The bladder samples were sent to be processed, blocked and sectioned to 8 μm at the University College London pathology lab. Once received, the slides were blinded with tape and numbered so that corresponding sections could be compared between bladders.

Immunohistochemical staining was performed using an avidin–biotin–peroxidase protocol as previously described [18,58]. Sections to be incubated with the anti-SNAP-25 antibody did not receive antigen retrieval, whereas those to be stained with the anti-cleaved SNAP-25 (anti-cSNAP-25) antibody were immersed in EDTA buffer (pH 9, Sigma-Aldrich, Gillingham, UK, E9884) at 98 °C. All sections were first blocked with 3% hydrogen peroxide (Sigma-Aldrich, Gillingham, UK, 1.07209), followed by 10% horse serum (Sigma-Aldrich, H1270) in Dako buffer. The sections were incubated at room temperature for one hour with anti-SNAP-25 (rabbit, 1/1000, Sigma-Aldrich, Gillingham, UK, S9684) and overnight with anti-cSNAP-25 (rabbit, 1/1000, provided by the research Pathology & Safety Biomarker Department, Ipsen Bioinnovation, Les Ulis, France). All sections (both primary antibodies) were incubated with a secondary biotinylated antibody (horse, 1/400, Vector Labs, Peterbrough, UK, BA-1100) for 30 min at room temperature. To amplify signals, Vectastain Elite ABC HRP Reagent (Vector Labs, PK-7100) was applied for 30 min at room temperature, followed by haematoxylin (Sigma-Aldrich, Gillingham, UK, H2126). Finally, slides were dehydrated with ethanol and xylene substitute Histochoice Clearing Agent (Sigma-Aldrich, Gillingham, UK, H2779). All slides were imaged using a light microscope, and the resulting image files were analysed in quadrants but not quantified, as preliminary analyses showed no cSNAP-25 staining in any of the bladders tested.

6. Patents

WO 2022/208091.

Supplementary Materials: The following supporting information can be downloaded at https://www.mdpi.com/article/10.3390/toxins16010030/s1. Figure S1: Negative and positive controls for total SNAP25 and cleaved SNAP-25 antibodies using skeletal muscle tissues sections from rats treated with aboBoNT-A.

Author Contributions: Conceptualisation D.M.D., J.M. and M.B.; methodology, D.M.D., H.I. and K.R.; formal analysis, H.I.; writing—original draft preparation, H.I., D.M.D., M.B. and J.M.; supervision, D.M.D., F.H. and M.B. All authors have read and agreed to the published version of the manuscript.

Funding: This research was funded by IPSEN bio innovation.

Institutional Review Board Statement: Experiments performed were in accordance with the ethical approval obtained from the UCLan Animal Welfare and Ethics Review Board (AWERB) (reference RE/16/11) (approval date: May 2017).

Informed Consent Statement: Not applicable.

Data Availability Statement: Datasets can be made available on request from the authors.

Conflicts of Interest: K.R., F.H., J.M. and M.B. were all employees of Ipsen at the time of this study.

References

1. Montecucco, C.; Molgó, J. Botulinal neurotoxins: Revival of an old killer. *Curr. Opin. Pharmacol.* **2005**, *5*, 274–279. [CrossRef] [PubMed]
2. Guyton, A.C.; MacDonald, M.A. Physiology of botulinus toxin. *Arch. Neurol. Psychiatry* **1947**, *57*, 578–592. [CrossRef] [PubMed]
3. Multani, I.; Manji, J.; Hastings-Ison, T.; Khot, A.; Graham, K. Botulinum toxin in the management of children with cerebral palsy *Pediatr. Drugs* **2019**, *21*, 261–281. [CrossRef] [PubMed]
4. Nestor, M.S.; Arnold, D.; Fischer, D. The mechanisms of action and use of botulinum neurotoxin type A in aesthetics: Key Clinical Postulates II. *J. Cosmet. Dermatol.* **2020**, *19*, 2785–2804. [CrossRef] [PubMed]
5. Abrams, P. Describing bladder storage function: Overactive bladder syndrome and detrusor overactivity. *Urology* **2003**, *62* (Suppl S2), 28–37; discussion 40–42. [CrossRef] [PubMed]
6. Reynolds, W.S.; Dmochowski, R.; Wein, A.; Bruehl, S. Does central sensitization help explain idiopathic overactive bladder? *Nat Rev. Urol.* **2016**, *13*, 481–491. [CrossRef] [PubMed]
7. Chapple, C.; Sievert, K.D.; MacDiarmid, S.; Khullar, V.; Radziszewski, P.; Nardo, C.; Thompson, C.; Zhou, J.; Haag-Molkenteller C. OnabotulinumtoxinA 100 U significantly improves all idiopathic overactive bladder symptoms and quality of life in patients with overactive bladder and urinary incontinence: A randomised, double-blind, placebo-controlled trial. *Eur. Urol.* **2013**, *64* 249–256. [CrossRef]
8. Chuang, Y.C.; Kaufmann, J.H.; Chancellor, D.D.; Chancellor, M.B.; Kuo, H.C. Bladder instillation of liposome encapsulated onabotulinumtoxina improves overactive bladder symptoms: A prospective, multicenter, double-blind, randomized trial. *J. Urol* **2014**, *192*, 1743–1749. [CrossRef]
9. Craciun, M.; Irwin, P. Outcomes for intravesical abobotulinumtoxin A (Dysport) treatment in the active management of overactive bladder symptoms—A prospective study. *Urology* **2019**, *130*, 54–58. [CrossRef]
10. Dmochowski, R.; Chapple, C.; Nitti, V.W.; Chancellor, M.; Everaert, K.; Thompson, C.; Daniell, G.; Zhou, J.; Haag-Molkenteller, C Efficacy and safety of onabotulinumtoxinA for idiopathic overactive bladder: A double-blind, placebo controlled, randomized dose ranging trial. *J. Urol.* **2010**, *184*, 2416–2422. [CrossRef]
11. Kuo, H.C.; Liu, H.T.; Chuang, Y.C.; Birder, L.A.; Chancellor, M.B. Pilot study of liposome-encapsulated onabotulinumtoxina fo patients with overactive bladder: A single-center study. *Eur. Urol.* **2014**, *65*, 1117–1124. [CrossRef] [PubMed]
12. Collins, V.M.; Daly, D.M.; Liaskos, M.; McKay, N.G.; Sellers, D.; Chapple, C.; Grundy, D. Onabotulinumtoxin A significantly attenuates bladder afferent nerve firing and inhibits ATP release from the urothelium. *BJU Int.* **2013**, *112*, 1018–1026. [CrossRef [PubMed]
13. Cui, M.; Khanijou, S.; Rubino, J.; Aoki, K.R. Subcutaneous administration of botulinum toxin A reduces formalin-induced pair *Pain* **2004**, *107*, 125–133. [CrossRef] [PubMed]
14. Favre-Guilmard, C.; Auguet, M.; Chabrier, E. Different antinociceptive effects of botulinum toxin type A in inflammatory an peripheral polyneuropathic rat models. *Eur. J. Pharmacol.* **2009**, *617*, 48–53. [CrossRef] [PubMed]
15. Burstein, R.; Zhang, X.; Levy, D.; Aoki, K.R.; Brin, M.F. Selective inhibition of meningeal nociceptors by botulinum neurotoxir type A: Therapeutic implications for migraine and other pains. *Cephalalgia* **2014**, *34*, 853–869. [CrossRef] [PubMed]
16. Zhang, X.; Strassman, A.M.; Novack, V.; Brin, M.F.; Burstein, R. Extracranial injections of botulinum neurotoxin type A inhibi intracranial meningeal nociceptors' responses to stimulation of TRPV1 and TRPA1 channels: Are we getting closer to solving thi puzzle? *Cephalalgia* **2016**, *36*, 875–886. [CrossRef]
17. Shone, C.; Agostini, H.; Clancy, J.; Gu, M.; Yang, H.; Chu, Y.; Johnson, V.; Taal, M.; McGlashan, J.; Brehm, J.; et al. Bivalent Recom binant Vaccine for Botulinum Neurotoxin Types A and B Based on a Polypeptide Comprising Their Effector and Translocatio Domains That Is Protective against the Predominant A and B Subtypes. *Infect. Immun.* **2009**, *77*, 2795–2801. [CrossRef]
18. Périer, C.; Martin, V.; Cornet, S.; Favre-Guilmard, C.; Rocher, M.N.; Bindler, J.; Wagner, S.; Andriambeloson, E.; Rudkin, B.B Marty, R.; et al. Recombinant botulinum neurotoxin serotype A1 in vivo characterization. *Pharmacol. Res. Perspect.* **2021**, *9*, e0085 [CrossRef]
19. Manecksha, R.P.; Cullen, I.M.; Ahmad, S.; McNeill, G.; Flynn, R.; McDermott, T.E.; Grainger, R.; Thornhill, J.A. Prospectiv randomised controlled trial comparing trigone-sparing versus trigone-including intradetrusor injection of abobotulinumtoxin for refractory idiopathic detrusor overactivity. *Eur. Urol.* **2012**, *61*, 928–935. [CrossRef]
20. Chuang, Y.C.; Tyagi, P.; Huang, C.C.; Yoshimura, N.; Wu, M.; Kaufman, J.; Chancellor, M.B. Urodynamic and immunohistochem cal evaluation of intravesical botulinum toxin A delivery using liposomes. *J. Urol.* **2009**, *182*, 786–792. [CrossRef]
21. Coelho, A.; Cruz, F.; Cruz, C.D.; Avelino, A. Spread of onabotulinumtoxinA after bladder injection. Experimental study using th distribution of cleaved SNAP-25 as the marker of the toxin action. *Eur. Urol.* **2012**, *61*, 1178–1184. [CrossRef]
22. Coelho, A.; Dinis, P.; Pinto, R.; Gorgal, T.; Silva, C.; Silva, A.; Silva, J.; Cruz, C.D.; Cruz, F.; Avelino, A. Distribution of th high-affinity binding site and intracellular target of botulinum toxin type A in the human bladder. *Eur. Urol.* **2010**, *57*, 884–89 [CrossRef] [PubMed]
23. Schiavo, G.G.; Benfenati, F.; Poulain, B.; Rossetto, O.; de Laureto, P.; DasGupta, B.R.; Montecucco, C. Tetanus and botulinum neurotoxins block neurotransmitter release by proteolytic cleavage of synaptobrevin. *Nature* **1992**, *359*, 832–835. [CrossRe [PubMed]

4. Baskaran, P.; Lehmann, T.E.; Topchiy, E.; Thirunavukkarasu, N.; Cai, S.; Singh, B.R.; Deshpande, S.; Thyagarajan, B. Effects of enzymatically inactive recombinant botulinum neurotoxin type A at the mouse neuromuscular junctions. *Toxicon* **2013**, *72*, 71–80. [CrossRef] [PubMed]
5. Li, L.; Binz, T.; Niemann, H.; Singh, B.R. Probing the mechanistic role of glutamate residue in the zinc-binding motif of type A botulinum neurotoxin light chain. *Biochemistry* **2000**, *39*, 2399–2405. [CrossRef]
6. Kukreja, R.V.; Sharma, S.; Cai, S.; Singh, B.R. Role of two active site Glu residues in the molecular action of botulinum neurotoxin endopeptidase. *Biochim. Et Biophys. Acta (BBA)-Proteins Proteom.* **2007**, *1774*, 213–222. [CrossRef]
7. Ravichandran, E.; Janardhanan, P.; Patel, K.; Riding, S.; Cai, S.; Singh, B.R. In vivo toxicity and immunological characterization of detoxified recombinant botulinum neurotoxin type A. *Pharm. Res.* **2016**, *33*, 639–652. [CrossRef]
8. Banerjee, A.; Li, G.; Alexander, E.A.; Schwartz, J.H. Role of SNAP-23 in trafficking of H+-ATPase in cultured inner medullary collecting duct cells. *Am. J. Physiol.-Cell Physiol.* **2001**, *280*, C775–C781. [CrossRef]
9. Vaidyanathan, V.V.; Yoshino, K.I.; Jahnz, M.; Dörries, C.; Bade, S.; Nauenburg, S.; Niemann, H.; Binz, T. Proteolysis of SNAP-25 isoforms by botulinum neurotoxin types A, C, and E: Domains and amino acid residues controlling the formation of enzyme-substrate complexes and cleavage. *J. Neurochem.* **1999**, *72*, 327–337. [CrossRef]
0. Hanna-Mitchell, A.T.; Wolf-Johnston, A.S.; Barrick, S.R.; Kanai, A.J.; Chancellor, M.B.; de Groat, W.C.; Birder, L.A. Effect of botulinum toxin A on urothelial-release of ATP and expression of SNARE targets within the urothelium. *Neurourol. Urodyn.* **2015**, *34*, 79–84. [CrossRef]
1. Birder, L.A.; Apodaca, G.; De Groat, W.C.; Kanai, A.J. Adrenergic-and capsaicin-evoked nitric oxide release from urothelium and afferent nerves in urinary bladder. *Am. J. Physiol.-Ren. Physiol.* **1998**, *275*, F226–F229. [CrossRef]
2. Ferguson, D.R.; Kennedy, I.; Burton, T. ATP is released from rabbit urinary bladder epithelial cells by hydrostatic pressure changes--a possible sensory mechanism? *J. Physiol.* **1997**, *505 Pt 2*, 503. [CrossRef]
3. Gillespie, J.I.; Markerink-van Ittersum, M.; De Vente, J. Expression of neuronal nitric oxide synthase (nNOS) and nitric-oxide-induced changes in cGMP in the urothelial layer of the guinea pig bladder. *Cell Tissue Res.* **2005**, *321*, 341–351. [CrossRef] [PubMed]
4. Olgart, C.; Gustafsson, L.E.; Wiklund, N.P. Evidence for nonvesicular nitric oxide release evoked by nerve activation. *Eur. J. Neurosci.* **2000**, *12*, 1303–1309. [CrossRef] [PubMed]
5. Ikeda, Y.; Zabbarova, I.V.; Birder, L.A.; de Groat, W.C.; McCarthy, C.J.; Hanna-Mitchell, A.T.; Kanai, A.J. Botulinum neurotoxin serotype A suppresses neurotransmitter release from afferent as well as efferent nerves in the urinary bladder. *Eur. Urol.* **2012**, *62*, 1157–1164. [CrossRef] [PubMed]

Beckel, J.M.; Daugherty, S.L.; Tyagi, P.; Wolf-Johnston, A.S.; Birder, L.A.; Mitchell, C.H.; de Groat, W.C. Pannexin 1 channels mediate the release of ATP into the lumen of the rat urinary bladder. *J. Physiol.* **2015**, *593*, 1857–1871. [CrossRef] [PubMed]

7. Silberfeld, A.; Chavez, B.; Obidike, C.; Daugherty, S.; de Groat, W.C.; Beckel, J.M. LPS-mediated release of ATP from urothelial cells occurs by lysosomal exocytosis. *Neurourol. Urodyn.* **2020**, *39*, 1321–1329. [CrossRef]

Ueda, N.; Kondo, M.; Takezawa, K.; Kiuchi, H.; Sekii, Y.; Inagaki, Y.; Soda, T.; Fukuhara, S.; Fujita, K.; Uemura, M.; et al. Bladder urothelium converts bacterial lipopolysaccharide information into neural signaling via an ATP-mediated pathway to enhance the micturition reflex for rapid defense. *Sci. Rep.* **2010**, *10*, 21167. [CrossRef]

Aizawa, N.; Igawa, Y.; Nishizawa, O.; Wyndaele, J.J. Effects of nitric oxide on the primary bladder afferent activities of the rat with and without intravesical acrolein treatment. *Eur. Urol.* **2011**, *59*, 264–271. [CrossRef]

Yu, Y.; de Groat, W.C. Nitric oxide modulates bladder afferent nerve activity in the in vitro urinary bladder–pelvic nerve preparation from rats with cyclophosphamide induced cystitis. *Brain Res.* **2013**, *1490*, 83–94. [CrossRef]

Argiolas, A.; Argiolas, F.M.; Argiolas, G.; Melis, M.R. Erectile Dysfunction: Treatments, Advances and New Therapeutic Strategies. *Brain Sci.* **2023**, *13*, 802. [CrossRef] [PubMed]

Rummel, A. Double receptor anchorage of botulinum neurotoxins accounts for their exquisite neurospecificity. *Botulinum Neurotoxins* **2013**, *364*, 61–90.

3. Chaddock, J.A.; Purkiss, J.R.; Friis, L.M.; Broadbridge, J.D.; Duggan, M.J.; Fooks, S.J.; Shone, C.C.; Quinn, C.P.; Foster, K.A. Inhibition of vesicular secretion in both neuronal and nonneuronal cells by a retargeted endopeptidase derivative of Clostridium botulinum neurotoxin type A. *Infect. Immun.* **2000**, *68*, 2587–2593. [CrossRef] [PubMed]

Jacky, B.P.; Garay, E.; Dupuy, J.; Nelson, J.B.; Cai, B.; Molina, Y.; Wang, J.; Steward, L.E.; Broide, R.S.; Francis, J.; et al. Identification of fibroblast growth factor receptor 3 (FGFR3) as a protein receptor for botulinum neurotoxin serotype A (BoNT/A). *PLoS Pathog.* **2013**, *9*, e1003369. [CrossRef]

James, N.G.; Malik, S.; Sanstrum, B.J.; Rhéaume, C.; Broide, R.S.; Jameson, D.M.; Brideau-Andersen, A.; Jacky, B.S. Characterization of clostridium botulinum neurotoxin serotype A (BoNT/A) and fibroblast growth factor receptor interactions using novel receptor dimerization assay. *Sci. Rep.* **2021**, *11*, 7832. [CrossRef] [PubMed]

Khandelwal, P.; Ruiz, W.G.; Balestreire-Hawryluk, E.; Weisz, O.A.; Goldenring, J.R.; Apodaca, G. Rab11a-dependent exocytosis of discoidal/fusiform vesicles in bladder umbrella cells. *Proc. Natl. Acad. Sci. USA* **2008**, *105*, 15773–15778. [CrossRef] [PubMed]

Clarke, H.; Soneji, N.; Ko, D.T.; Yun, L.; Wijeysundera, D.N. Rates and risk factors for prolonged opioid use after major surgery: Population based cohort study. *BMJ* **2014**, *348*, g1251. [CrossRef] [PubMed]

Stone, A.B.; Wick, E.C.; Wu, C.L.; Grant, M.C. The US opioid crisis: A role for enhanced recovery after surgery. *Anesth. Analg.* **2017**, *125*, 1803–1805. [CrossRef]

49. Field, M.; Splevins, A.; Picaut, P.; Schans, M.; Langenberg, J.; Noort, D.; Foster, K. AbobotulinumtoxinA (Dysport®), Onab tulinumtoxinA (Botox®), and IncobotulinumtoxinA (Xeomin®) Neurotoxin Content and Potential Implications for Duration c Response in Patients. *Toxins* **2018**, *10*, 535. [CrossRef]
50. Maignel-Ludop, J.; Huchet, M.; Krupp, J. Botulinum Neurotoxins Serotypes A and B induce paralysis of mouse striated an smooth muscles with different potencies. *Pharmacol. Res. Perspect.* **2017**, *5*, e00289. [CrossRef]
51. Daly, D.; Rong, W.; Chess-Williams, R.; Chapple, C.; Grundy, D. Bladder afferent sensitivity in wild-type and TRPV1 knockou mice. *J. Physiol.* **2007**, *583*, 663–674. [CrossRef] [PubMed]
52. Daly, D.M.; Chess-Williams, R.; Chapple, C.; Grundy, D. The inhibitory role of acetylcholine and muscarinic receptors in bladde afferent activity. *Eur. Urol.* **2010**, *58*, 22–28. [CrossRef] [PubMed]
53. Daly, D.M.; Nocchi, L.; Liaskos, M.; McKay, N.G.; Chapple, C.; Grundy, D. Age-related changes in afferent pathways an urothelial function in the male mouse bladder. *J. Physiol.* **2014**, *592*, 537–549. [CrossRef] [PubMed]
54. Grundy, L.; Erickson, A.; Caldwell, A.; Garcia-Caraballo, S.; Rychkov, G.; Harrington, A.; Brierley, S.M. Tetrodotoxin-sensitiv voltage-gated sodium channels regulate bladder afferent responses to distension. *Pain* **2018**, *159*, 2573–2584. [CrossRef] [PubMe
55. Konthapakdee, N.; Grundy, L.; O'Donnell, T.; Garcia-Caraballo, S.; Brierley, S.M.; Grundy, D.; Daly, D.M. Serotonin exerts a dire modulatory role on bladder afferent firing in mice. *J. Physiol.* **2019**, *597*, 5247–5264. [CrossRef]
56. Rong, W.; Spyer, K.M.; Burnstock, G. Activation and sensitisation of low and high threshold afferent fibres mediated by P2 receptors in the mouse urinary bladder. *J. Physiol.* **2002**, *541*, 591–600. [CrossRef]
57. Vlaskovska, M.; Kasakov, L.; Rong, W.; Bodin, P.; Bardini, M.; Cockayne, D.A.; Ford, A.P. Burnstock GP2X3 knock-out mice reve a major sensory role for urothelially released ATP. *J. Neurosci.* **2001**, *21*, 5670–5677. [CrossRef]
58. Retailleau, K.; Martin, V.; Lezmi, S.; Nicoleau, C.; Maignel, J. The isolated mouse jejunal afferent nerve assay as a tool to assess th effect of botulinum neurotoxins in visceral nociception. *Toxins* **2022**, *14*, 205. [CrossRef]

toxins

MDPI

Review

Strategies for Safe Transurethral Injections of Botulinum Toxin into the Bladder Wall

Matthias Oelke [1,2]

[1] Hannover Medical School, Siedlerweg 10, 48599 Gronau, Germany; dr.moelke@t-online.de; Tel.: +31-6-29-74-15-52
[2] Kantonsspital Frauenfeld, Spital Thurgau AG, Waldeggstr. 8A, 8500 Frauenfeld, Switzerland

Abstract: Introduction: Transurethral injections into the bladder wall with botulinum toxin are an established treatment for refractory overactive bladder or detrusor overactivity. With the current injection technique, an average of approx. 18% and up to 40% of botulinum toxin is injected next to the bladder wall, potentially causing reduced efficacy or non-response. The article aims to evaluate the reasons for incorrect injections and propose strategies for complete delivery of the entire botulinum toxin fluid into the bladder wall. **Material and Methods:** Unstructured literature search and narrative review of the literature. **Results:** Incorrect injection of botulinum toxin fluid next to the bladder wall is caused by pushing the injection needle too deep and through the bladder wall. Bladder wall thickness decreases with increasing bladder filling and has a thickness of less than 2 mm beyond 100 mL in healthy individuals. Ultrasound imaging of the bladder wall before botulinum toxin injection can verify bladder wall thickness in individual patients. Patient movements during the injection therapy increase the chance of incorrect placement of the needle tip. **Conclusions:** Based on the literature search, it is helpful and recommended to (1) perform pretreatment ultrasound imaging of the bladder to estimate bladder wall thickness and to adjust the injection depth accordingly, (2) fill the bladder as low as possible, ideally below 100 mL, (3) use short needles, ideally 2 mm, and (4) provide sufficient anesthesia and pain management to avoid patient movements during the injection therapy.

Keywords: botulinum toxin; overactive bladder; detrusor overactivity; neurogenic bladder dysfunction; detrusor wall thickness; injection

Key Contribution: For complete injection of the botulinum toxin fluid into the bladder wall, it is essential to know bladder wall thickness, fill the bladder with saline solution as low as possible, use short injection needles, and use sufficient anesthesia to avoid patient movements.

1. Introduction

Transurethral injections of botulinum toxin into the bladder wall are a recommended and well-accepted treatment option for female or male patients with treatment-refractory overactive bladder or (neurogenic or non-neurogenic) detrusor overactivity with or without urinary urgency incontinence [1–4]. Therefore, transurethral botulinum toxin injections should be considered when previous treatments have failed, such as conservative treatment (e.g., behavioral modifications, lifestyle advice), pelvic floor muscle exercise with or without biofeedback, drug treatment with muscarinic receptor antagonists and/or β_3-adrenoceptor agonists, and electrostimulation. Although not licensed for this indication, botulinum toxin may also be applied as a fourth-line treatment for interstitial cystitis/bladder pain syndrome, as recommended by the AUA guidelines [5,6].

Botulinum toxin is a bacterial neurotoxin with 1296 amino acids and a molecular weight of 146 kDa produced by several *clostridium* species, of which *clostridium botulinum*, *clostridium butyricum*, *clostridium baratii*, or *clostridium argentinense* are the most important [7]. Of the seven known subtypes of botulinum toxin, only types A and B are commercially available, of which onabotulinum toxin A since 2013 (Botox®; Allergan Pharmaceuticals, Dublin,

Ireland) and abobotulinum toxin A since 2022 (Dysport®; Ipsen, Boulogne-Billancourt, France) are licensed for the treatment of overactive bladder or (neurogenic) detrusor overactivity. In comparison, Botox® has a total molecular weight of approx. 900 kDa (146 kDa neurotoxin + approx. 750 kDa protein chains) and Dysport® has a molecular weight of approx. 500 kDa (146 kDa neurotoxin + approx. 350 kDa protein chains) [8]. Botulinum toxin from both companies is stored as white crystalline powder (lyophilizates) in vacuum-sealed glass bottles and must be dissolved in sterile saline solution before use. Because of the high molecular weight of both botulinum toxin formulations and the impermeable urothelial layer, botulinum toxin must be injected into the bladder wall to reach the target tissue, i.e., the parasympathetic nerve terminals of the detrusor and/or submucosa, thereby inhibiting acetylcholine release into the synaptic cleft [9] and, finally, decreasing bladder sensations as well as detrusor muscle contractions [10]. Submucosal injections of botulinum toxin have been shown to be as effective as intradetrusor injections [11]. Consequently, the botulinum toxin solution must be injected into the submucosal layer and/or detrusor, whereas injections outside these tissue layers (perivesical space) do not reach the parasympathetic nerve terminals and, therefore, do not show clinical effects.

Mehnert et al. noted that a standardization of the injection technique is still missing and, with the help of magnetic resonance imaging (MRI) and contrast media, demonstrated that an average of approx. 18% of the injected botulinum toxin solution was eventually injected into the perivesical fatty tissue (average of 53 U of the 300 U Botox®) [12]. The authors investigated six adult patients aged 18 to 82 years with neurogenic detrusor overactivity incontinence due to spinal cord injury at levels Th6 to Th11. They used rigid cystoscopes and 22G needles with a length of 8 mm, which were retracted by approx. half of the length (i.e., 4 mm) after pricking the bladder wall at the dome and base. Immediately after the injections, MRI was performed, the contrast media inside and outside the bladder wall visualized, and the volume of contrast media in both locations calculated. In men, 8.2–15.9 cm^3 (14.6%) of the injected contrast media was detected lateral of bladder walls (i.e., 44 U Botox®) and, in women, 2.5–14.4 cm^3 (20.8%; i.e., 62 U Botox®). One female patient had spastic limb contractions during the operation, and the injection procedure with withdrawing the needle by approx. half of the length for bladder wall injections was more difficult; consequently, 40% of the total injected contrast media solution was located lateral of the bladder walls (120 U Botox®). The majority of perivesical contrast media was seen lateral to the bladder dome and, in one patient, beyond the bladder base. Unfortunately, the authors did not report on the bladder filling volume during the botulinum toxin injections.

Based on the results of this study, it becomes evident that perivesical injections of botulinum toxin were caused by pushing the tip of the injection needle through the bladder wall. Although the needle was retracted by approx. half of its length (4 mm), this maneuver did not prevent false injections. The question arises: how deep can the injection needle be inserted into the bladder wall to safely deliver the total botulinum toxin fluid to the target location? This article deals with theoretical and practical considerations of the injection technique for safe delivery of (nearly) 100% of the botulinum toxin dose into the bladder wall.

2. Bladder Wall Thickness in Relation to Bladder Filling Volume

The bladder wall can be imaged well with high-frequency ultrasound probes (e.g., 7.5 MHz) by the suprapubic or transrectal route in men as well as the suprapubic, transrectal, transvaginal, or transperineal route in women [13,14]. The technique of ultrasound detrusor wall thickness (DWT) measurements has been described earlier [15]. The mucosa and adventitia of the bladder wall appear hyperechogenic (white), while the detrusor in between these two layers appears hypoechogenic (black, Figure 1) [14,16,17]. Initial studies in healthy, young adult women and men focused on the relationship between bladder/detrusor wall thickness and bladder filling volume and demonstrated a decreasing thickness with increasing bladder filling [17]. In this study, detrusor wall thickness (DWT) was measured every 50 mL until 300 mL of bladder filling volume and, afterwards, every

100 mL until maximum bladder capacity. The study showed in both women and men a rapidly decreasing DWT during the bladder filling until approx. 100 mL and a slower decrease until bladder capacity (Figure 2). DWT was measured at approx. 2.5–4.5 mm at low bladder filling and reached an average DWT of 1.2 mm (women) to 1.4 mm (men) at capacity.

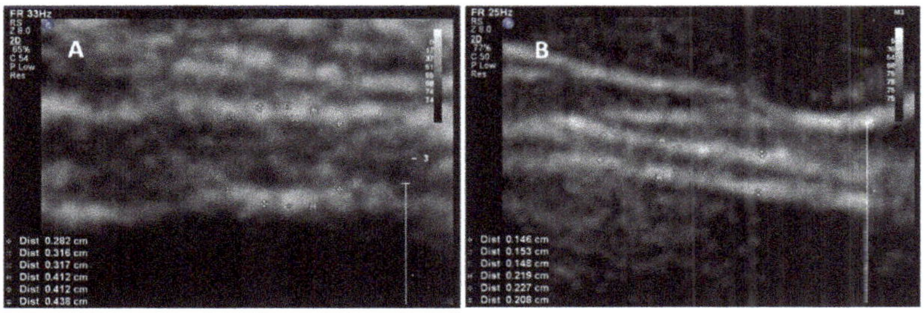

Figure 1. Imaging of the anterior bladder wall with a suprapubically positioned ultrasound probe in a patient aged 46 years with overactive bladder/detrusor overactivity, both images 6-times enlarged. The detrusor appears hypoechogenic (black) and is sandwiched between the mucosa and adventitia, which both appear hyperechogenic (white). The detrusor (upper three measurements, i.e., detrusor wall thickness) and the entire bladder wall (lower three measurements, i.e., bladder wall thickness) were measured. (**A**) Bladder wall of the bladder filled with 50 mL and (**B**) with 250 mL (source: private image collection M. Oelke).

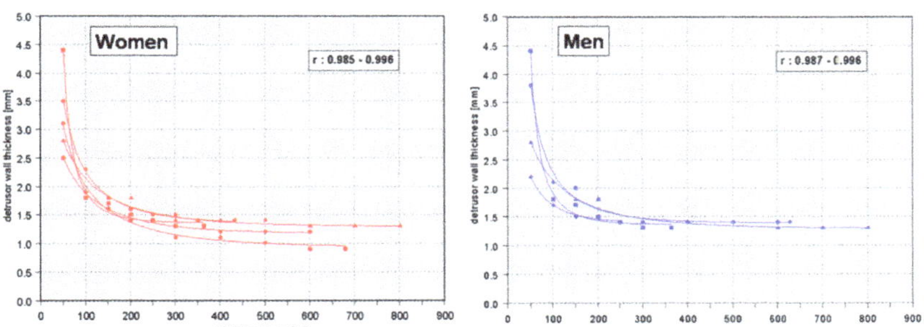

Figure 2. Relationship between bladder filling (x-axis) and detrusor wall thickness (y-axis) in four different healthy women (**left**) and four healthy men (**right**). Measurements of the same person at different bladder fillings were connected with lines. Detrusor wall thickness rapidly decreases during the first 100–150 mL of bladder filling but only decreases slightly thereafter [17].

This study on the relationship between DWT and bladder filling shows that it is crucial to know and control the bladder filling volume during botulinum toxin injections. Consequently, botulinum toxin fluid is correctly and completely delivered into the bladder wall when the physician uses a short needle and the bladder is only filled with a low volume (e.g., 50–100 mL), whereas the needle with the same length is pushed through the entire bladder wall and botulinum toxin fluid is injected outside the bladder wall when the bladder is filled with a higher volume (e.g., 300–400 mL).

3. Adjustments to the Injection Technique

The author of this current article modifies his injection technique by pretreatment ultrasound imaging of the bladder wall in all patients because bladder wall thickness, compared to healthy individuals, can be increased in patients with bladder outlet obstruction [15,18] (Figure 3) as well as in some patients with neurogenic bladder dysfunction (e.g., low compliance due to myelomeningocele/spina bifida or paraplegia) [19,20] or decreased in patients with detrusor underactivity [21]. Routine ultrasound imaging of the bladder wall provides useful information about how deep the needle can be inserted into the bladder wall for safe delivery of the entire botulinum toxin fluid, especially in patients with suspected thinner bladder walls, e.g., younger patients (children or teenagers), women, and those with suspicion of detrusor underactivity.

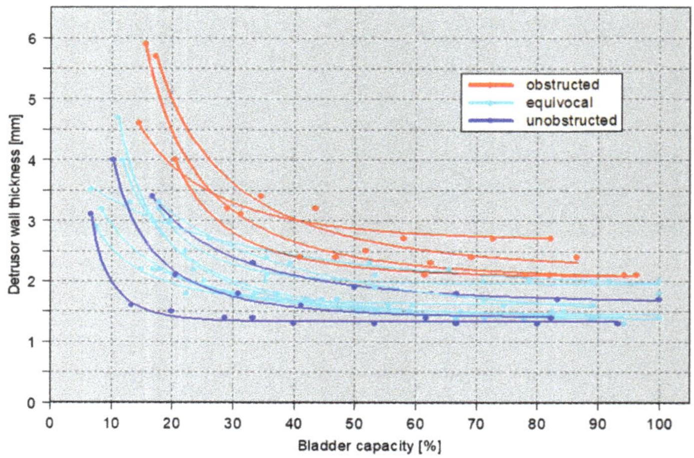

Figure 3. Relationship between bladder capacity (*x*-axis) and detrusor wall thickness (*y*-axis) in men with benign prostatic hyperplasia: without (dark blue), equivocal (light blue), and with bladder outlet obstruction (red). In contrast to Figure 2, bladder filling (ml) was changed to % bladder capacity to adjust for the differences in bladder capacity in the individual patients. Measurements of the same person at different bladder fillings were connected with lines. Like healthy individuals, detrusor wall thickness rapidly decreases during the first phase of bladder filling but only slightly thereafter. The extent of bladder wall hypertrophy (detrusor wall thickness) is dependent on the degree of bladder outlet obstruction (source: private image collection, M. Oelke).

The injection technique must be further modified when using rigid cystoscopes because the bladder dome (cranial part of the bladder) is usually penetrated by the needle in a perpendicular (orthograde) fashion, whereas the lateral bladder walls and the bladder base are usually penetrated in a tangential direction, the latter locations providing a longer distance of the injection route (Figure 4). Therefore, the author of this current article fills the bladder only with low volume (<100 mL), uses 4 mm needles that are retracted by approx. half of their length (2 mm) after pricking the bladder wall and before injection of the botulinum toxin fluid, and prefers tangential injections wherever possible.

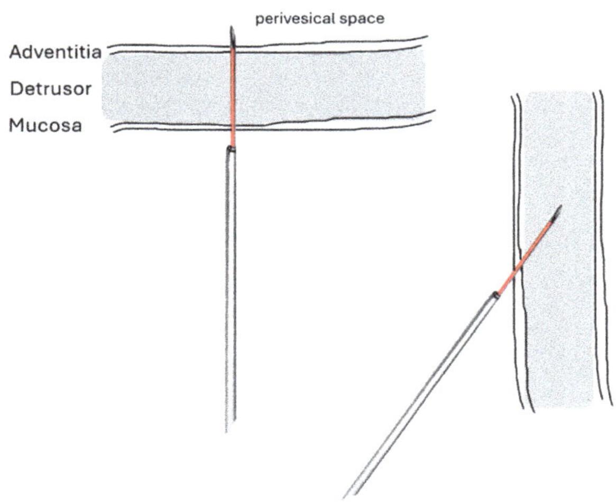

Figure 4. Illustration of perpendicular (e.g., at the bladder dome) and tangential insertion of the injection needle (e.g., at the lateral bladder wall or bladder base). In this figure, a needle length of 4 mm was chosen. Tangential insertion provides a longer distance within the bladder wall and, therefore, a higher chance to inject botulinum toxin at the correct location (source: private image collection, M. Oelke).

4. Discussion

The authors of the MRI-based study demonstrated that an average of 18% (and up to 40%) of the botulinum injection fluid was delivered next (laterally) to the bladder after pricking the bladder wall and inserting the needle by approx. 4 mm [12]. Their study was conducted in patients with paraplegia who usually have thickened bladder walls due to the underlying disease [19,20]. It can be hypothesized that a larger and more substantial amount of botulinum toxin fluid would have been injected beyond the bladder wall when using the identical injection technique and treating patients without thickened bladder walls (e.g., women with non-neurogenic overactive bladder). This may be one reason why transurethral botulinum toxin treatment remains ineffective in some patients.

For safe and complete delivery of the botulinum toxin fluid into the bladder wall, it is important to minimize the bladder filling, which, however, should be high enough to see all parts of the bladder during the procedure. This situation is usually achieved when the bladder has been filled with 50–100 mL. The penetration depth of the needle should also be adjusted to the location of the bladder wall injections (dome vs. lateral walls). The shorter the needle or the lower the penetration depth of the needle, the higher the chance of correct and complete injections of botulinum toxin fluid. The industry has lately provided short needles for this purpose (e.g., injeTAK® cystoscopy needles with an adjustable injection depth between 2 and 5 mm with 1 mm increments; Laborie, Portsmouth, NH, USA). These needles must not be retracted after pricking of the bladder wall, especially when bladder wall thickness is known in the individual patient by ultrasound investigation before the procedure. Although superficial injections are more likely with these needles, previous studies and a meta-analysis have shown similar efficacy of submucosal vs. intradetrusor injections [11]. Submucosal injections can be visualized by bulking of the mucosa into the bladder lumen at the injection site, whereas this bulking is missing with intradetrusor (or perivesical) injections.

Adequate anesthesia for painless injections is another factor contributing to the correct placement of the botulinum toxin dose into the bladder wall. It was demonstrated in the study by Mehnert et al. that patient movements during pricking of the bladder wall and/or retracting the needle before the injections can result in perivesical placement of the botulinum toxin solution of up to 40% of the total injected dose [12]. Sufficient anesthesia of the bladder can be achieved by transurethral instillation of (alkalized) lidocaine or related anesthetics, regional, or general anesthesia. Local anesthesia has the advantage of avoiding the presence of anesthesiologists, intra- and postoperative screening of the patient's vital parameters, and anesthesia-related risks. The author of this current article has been using local anesthesia for the last 4 years in approx. 300 patients without or only minimal pain (visual analog pain 0–2 on a Likert scale reaching from 0 to 10). He uses transurethral bladder installations with 50 mL lidocaine 2% in combination with 50 mL sodium bicarbonate 8.4% at a temperature of approx. 5 °C (refrigerator) 20 to 30 min before the botulinum toxin injection treatment. Pereira e Silva et al. demonstrated in a double-blind, randomized, controlled study that lidocaine and sodium bicarbonate together significantly decrease pain scores better than lidocaine alone [22]. Immediately before cystoscopy and bladder wall injections, the author of this current article additionally injects half (women) or one syringe (men) with 11 mL lidocaine-chlorhexidine gel (InstillaGel®; Farco Pharma, Cologne, Germany) at a temperature of approx. 5 °C (refrigerator) into the urethra for lubrication, disinfection, and anesthesia. Electromotive drug administration (EMDA) with lidocaine 4% has also been shown to significantly decrease pain during botulinum toxin injections compared to lidocaine instillations alone [23]. In rare cases, reduction in the injection sites (without decreasing the total botulinum toxin dose) [24,25] or oral phenazopyridine, which is excreted via the kidneys and has a local anesthetic effect on the urinary tract, can also significantly reduce pain during botulinum toxin treatment [26].

Intravesical instillation of liposome-encapsulated botulinum toxin A (lipo-botulinum toxin) could overcome the issues of perivesical injections, bladder filling, and pain management in the future. Liposomes are small lipophile two-layer phospholipid vesicles that can fuse with cell membranes, pass the usually impermeable urothelial layer, and release the content of the aqueous core with botulinum toxin for safe delivery of the drug into the target tissue in the submucosa or detrusor [27,28]. Despite promising pilot studies, lipo-botulinum toxin has not yet become commercially available.

5. Conclusions

Physicians aim to inject the intended botulinum toxin dose completely into the bladder wall, thereby avoiding perivesical injections and reducing the clinical effects. A summary of the methods supporting complete injection of the botulinum toxin fluid is visualized in Figure 5. Preoperative visualization of the bladder wall helps judge bladder wall thickness in individual patients. Because bladder wall thickness decreases with increasing bladder filling volume, it is necessary to fill the bladder as low as possible but high enough to see all parts of the bladder. This situation is usually achieved when the bladder has been filled with a physiological saline solution of <100 mL. In addition, physicians should use short needles (e.g., 2 mm) for safe injections of the botulinum toxin fluid into the submucosal layer of the bladder and/or detrusor. Adequate pain management during the injection therapy (e.g., lidocaine-sodium bicarbonate instillations 20–30 min before) further contributes to the safe and predictable application of botulinum toxin. The proposed strategies are important for predictable, reliable, and reproducible clinical results, especially during re-injections and up- or down-titration of the botulinum toxin dose in patients with too low or too large effects during the first botulinum toxin treatment(s).

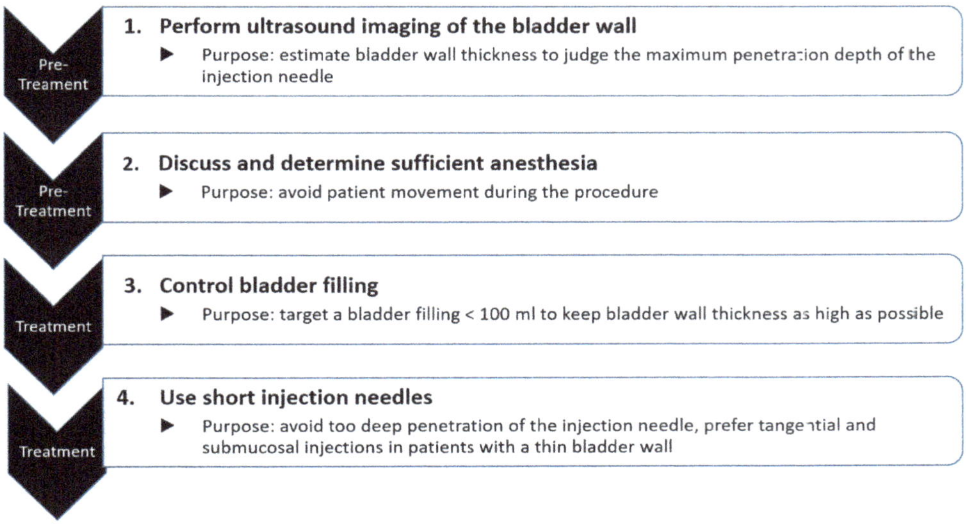

Figure 5. Summary of the four methods to minimize the chance of perivesical injections of botulinum toxin fluid into the bladder wall.

Funding: This research received no external funding.

Institutional Review Board Statement: Not applicable.

Informed Consent Statement: Not applicable.

Data Availability Statement: Not applicable.

Conflicts of Interest: The author declares no conflict of interest.

eferences

Nambiar, A.K.; Arlandis, S.; Bø, K.; Cobussen-Boekhorst, H.; Costantini, E.; de Heide, M.; Farag, F.; Groen, J.; Karavitakis, M.; Lapitan, M.C.; et al. European Association of Urology guidelines on the diagnosis and management of female non-neurogenic lower urinary tract symptoms. Part 1: Diagnostics, overactive bladder, stress urinary incontinence, and mixed urinary incontinence. *Eur. Urol.* **2022**, *82*, 49–59. [CrossRef] [PubMed]

Gacci, M.; Sakalis, V.I.; Karavitakis, M.; Cornu, J.N.; Gratzke, C.; Herrmann, T.R.; Kyriazis, I.; Malde, S.; Mamoulakis, C.; Rieken, M.; et al. European Association of Urology guidelines on male urinary incontinence. *Eur. Urol.* **2022**, *82*, 387–398. [CrossRef] [PubMed]

Sartori, A.M.; Kessler, T.M.; Castro-Díaz, D.M.; de Keijzer, P.; Del Popolo, G.; Ecclestone, H.; Frings, D.; Groen, J.; Hamid, R.; Karsenty, G.; et al. Summary of the 2024 update of the European Association of Urology guidelines on neurourology. *Eur. Urol.* **2024**, *85*, 543–555. [CrossRef] [PubMed]

Naumann, G.; Aigmüller, T.; Bader, W.; Bauer, R.; Beilecke, K.; Meier, C.B.; Bruer, G.; Bschleipfer, T.; Deniz, M.; Fink, T.; et al. Diagnosis and Therapy of Female Urinary Incontinence. Guideline of the DGGG, OEGGG and SGGG (S2k Level, AWMF Registry No. 015/091, January 2022): Part 2 with recommendations on interventional/surgical therapy of overactive bladder, surgical treatment of stress urinary incontinence and diagnosis and therapy of iatrogenic urogenital fistula. *Geburtshilfe Frauenheilkd.* **2023**, *83*, 410–436. [PubMed]

Hanno, P.M.; Erickson, D.; Moldwin, R.; Faraday, M.M. Diagnosis and treatment of interstitial cystitis/bladder pain syndrome: AUA guideline amendment. *J. Urol.* **2015**, *193*, 1545–1553. [CrossRef] [PubMed]

Jiang, Y.H.; Jhang, J.F.; Kuo, H.C. The clinical application of intravesical botulinum toxin A injection in patients with overactive bladder and interstitial cystitis. *Tzu Chi Med. J.* **2023**, *35*, 31–37.

Popoff, M.R.; Bouvet, P. Genetic characteristics of toxigenic clostridia and toxin gene evolution. *Toxicon* **2013**, *75*, 63–89. [CrossRef] [PubMed]

Aoki, K.R.; Guyer, B. Botulinum toxin type A and other botulinum toxin serotypes: A comparative review of biochemical and pharmacological actions. *Eur. J. Neurol.* **2001**, *8* (Suppl. S5), 21–29. [CrossRef] [PubMed]

9. Lin, Y.H.; Chiang, B.J.; Liao, C.H. Mechanism of action of botulinum toxin A in treatment of functional urological disorder *Toxins* **2020**, *12*, 129. [CrossRef]
10. Mangera, A.; Apostolidis, A.; Andersson, K.E.; Dasgupta, P.; Giannantoni, A.; Roehrborn, C.; Novara, G.; Chapple, C. An update systematic review and statistical comparison of standardized mean outcomes for the use of botulinum toxin in the managemer of lower urinary tract disorders. *Eur. Urol.* **2014**, *65*, 981–990. [CrossRef]
11. Li, G.P.; Wand, X.Y.; Zhang, Y. Efficacy and safety of onabotulinumtoxinA in patients with neurogenic detrusor overactivit caused by spinal cord injury: A systematic review and meta-analysis. *Int. Neurourol. J.* **2018**, *22*, 275–286. [CrossRef] [PubMed]
12. Mehnert, U.; Boy, S.; Schmid, M.; Reitz, A.; von Hessling, A.; Hodler, J.; Schurch, B. A morphological evaluation of botulinur neurotoxin A injections into the detrusor muscle using magnetic resonance imaging. *World J. Urol.* **2009**, *27*, 397–403. [CrossRe [PubMed]
13. Oelke, M.; Wijkstra, H. Ultrasound detrusor wall thickness measurements to diagnose bladder outlet obstruction in me *Urodinamica* **2006**, *16*, 343–352.
14. Oelke, M.; Khullar, V.; Wijkstra, H. Review on ultrasound measurement of bladder or detrusor wall thickness in wome Techniques, diagnostic utility, and use in clinical trials. *World J. Urol.* **2013**, *31*, 1093–1104. [CrossRef] [PubMed]
15. Oelke, M.; Höfner, K.; Wiese, B.; Grünewald, V.; Jonas, U. Increase in detrusor wall thickness indicates bladder outlet obstructic (BOO) in men. *World J. Urol.* **2002**, *19*, 443–452. [CrossRef] [PubMed]
16. Kojima, M.; Inui, E.; Ochiai, A.; Naya, Y.; Ukimura, O.; Watanabe, H. Ultrasonic estimation of bladder weight as a measure bladder hypertrophy in men with infravesical obstruction: A preliminary report. *Urology* **1996**, *47*, 942–947. [CrossRef] [PubMe
17. Oelke, M.; Höfner, K.; Jonas, U.; Ubbink, D.; de la Rosette, J.; Wijkstra, H. Ultrasound measurement of detrusor wall thickness i healthy adults. *Neururol. Urodyn.* **2006**, *25*, 308–317. [CrossRef] [PubMed]
18. Manieri, C.; Carter, S.S.C.; Romano, G.; Trucchi, A.; Valenti, M.; Tubaro, A. The diagnosis of bladder outlet obstruction in men b ultrasound measurement of bladder wall thickness. *J. Urol.* **1998**, *159*, 761–765. [CrossRef]
19. Ukimura, O.; Kojima, M.; Iwata, T.; Inaba, M.; Miki, T. Ultrasonic measurement of bladder weight as a novel urodynamic modali *Adv. Exp. Med. Biol.* **2003**, *539 Pt A*, 311–315.
20. Silva, J.A.F.; Gonsalves, M.D.C.D.; de Melo, R.T.; Carrerette, F.B.; Damião, R. Association between the bladder wall thickness an urodynamic findings in patients with spinal cord injury. *World J. Urol.* **2015**, *33*, 131–135. [CrossRef]
21. Rademakers, K.L.; van Koeveringe, G.A.; Oelke, M. Ultrasound detrusor wall thickness measurement in combination wi bladder capacity can safely detect detrusor underactivity in adult men. *World J. Urol.* **2017**, *35*, 153–159. [CrossRef] [PubMed]
22. Pereira e Silva, R.; Ponte, C.; Lopes, F.; Palma dos Reis, J. Alkalinized lidocaine solution as a first-line local anesthesia protocol f intradetrusor injection of onabotulinum toxin A: Results from a double-blinded randomized controlled trial. *Neurourol. Urody* **2020**, *39*, 2471–2479. [CrossRef] [PubMed]
23. Schurch, B.; Reitz, A.; Tenti, G. Electromotive drug administration of lidocaine to anesthetize the bladder before botulinum toxin injections into the detrusor. *Spinal Cord.* **2004**, *42*, 338–341. [CrossRef] [PubMed]
24. Lo, W.; Lo, M.C. Botulinum toxin-A (boNT/A) in the treatment of idiopathic detrusor overactivity (IDO) incontinence. prospective randomized study to compare 20 vs. 10 injection sites. *BJU Int.* **2015**, *116* (Suppl. S4), 1–27.
25. Briskin, R.; Atiemo, H. Evaluation of patient reported pain perception during office-based onabotulinumtoxina injection. *Neurour Urodyn.* **2021**, *40* (Suppl. S1), S6–S242.
26. Stewart, L.E.; Siddique, M.; Jacobs, K.M.; Raker, C.A.; Sung, V.W. Oral phenazopyridine vs intravesical lidocaine for bladd onabotulinumtoxinA analgesia: A randomized controlled trial. *Am J Obstet Gynecol.* **2022**, *227*, 308.e1–308.e8. [CrossRe [PubMed]
27. Chuang, Y.C.; Kaufmann, J.H.; Chancellor, D.D.; Chancellor, M.B.; Kuo, H.C. Bladder instillation of liposome encapsul onabotulinumtoxina improves overactive bladder symptoms: A prospective, multicenter, double-blind, randomized trial. *J. Ur* **2024**, *192*, 1743–1749. [CrossRef]
28. Hung, F.C.; Kuo, H.C. Liposome-encapsulated botulinum toxin A in treatment of functional bladder disorders. *Toxins* **20** *14*, 838. [CrossRef]

toxins

MDPI

Article

Efficacy, Satisfaction, and Compliance: Insights from 15 Years of Botulinum Toxin Use for Female Urgency Urinary Incontinence

Margarida Manso [1,2,*], João Diogo Soares [2], Margarida Henriques [1], Francisco Botelho [1,3], Carlos Silva [1,2] and Francisco Cruz [1,2]

1 Urology Department, Centro Hospitalar Universitário São João, 4200-319 Porto, Portugal
2 Faculdade de Medicina da Universidade do Porto, 4200-319 Porto, Portugal
3 Instituto de Investigação em Ciências da Vida e Saúde, Escola de Medicina da Universidade do Minho, 4710-057 Braga, Portugal
* Correspondence: manso.margarida@gmail.com

Abstract: Urgency urinary incontinence (UUI) refractory to medical treatment poses significant challenges despite advancements. This study evaluates the efficacy of intravesical botulinum toxin for UUI and identifies factors influencing treatment outcomes. Among 368 women receiving botulinum toxin injections, 74.5% achieved a complete discontinuation of pad usage. Predictors of efficacy included lower pre-treatment pad usage and the absence of prior sling placement. Patients often required repeat injections (60.3%), with younger age and satisfaction correlating with treatment repetition. The interval between injections averaged 18 months, influenced by logistical challenges and patient preferences. Despite concerns about diminishing efficacy, subjective perceptions did not align with objective findings. Limitations include retrospective analysis and heterogeneous clinical records. In conclusion, intravesical botulinum toxin is effective for UUI, with pre-treatment pad usage and sling placement history influencing outcomes and patient characteristics influencing treatment repetition.

Keywords: female urinary incontinence; urgency urinary incontinence; overactive bladder; bladder botulinum toxin; Botox®

Key Contribution: UUI treatment with botulinum toxin type A bladder injection maintains a long-term constant efficacy, and intervals between treatment cycles are wider than expected from pivotal trials. Patients with a more severe condition and a history of previous slings procedures should be informed about their lower likelihood of success.

1. Introduction

While urgency urinary incontinence (UUI) may not be the most common form of incontinence, it often prompts individuals to seek medical attention more frequently than other types. Most cases are idiopathic, and it is generally assumed to be associated with the aging process, although other risk factors are identified [1,2].

According to European Association of Urology guidelines, the first-line treatment of UUI, whether included or not in the overactive bladder (OAB) syndrome, relies on lifestyle interventions and bladder training, with second-line being pharmacotherapy. Anticholinergics have revolutionized the treatment of UUI, but the associated side effects and the need for continuous medication lead many patients to discontinue treatment. Despite valuable additions such as beta-3 agonists, a substantial number of cases either do not improve or show only limited progress. When pharmacotherapy fails or cannot be tolerated, a bladder wall injection of botulinum toxin is one of the third-line therapies [2,3].

However, it is essential to acknowledge that even with this therapy, there are both refractory patients and individuals who, over the long term, discontinue treatment despite initially positive responses. The reasons for such discontinuation remain unclear and cannot be determined by pivotal studies. Therefore, in this study, we aim to clarify if we can predict which patients will respond favorably or unfavorably, if there are factors influencing the efficacy and duration of the treatment, and which patients are more likely to request repeated injections, as well as the efficacy of botulinum toxin in treating UUI in real-life conditions.

2. Results

The study involved 368 women diagnosed with UUI between 2010 and the last quarter of 2023, all of whom underwent bladder injections of botulinum toxin. Patients injected after that date were not included due to the inability to properly analyze the duration of the treatment. Of the 368 patients analyzed, the mean age at diagnosis was 60.4 years (SD $\pm$ 14.1) and had an average BMI of 30.3 (SD $\pm$ 5.4). In this cohort, 27.7% had undergone a previous mid-urethral sling placement. Among those with available information, 67.7% had a transobturator tape, 25% had a single incision sling, and 7.3% had a retropubic sling.

Among the 306 patients with complete information concerning pad usage, the median number of pads used per day before botulinum toxin injection was 3 (p25–p75: 2–5), which subsequently decreased to 0 (p25–p75: 0–1) post injection. The majority (74.5%) of patients reported a complete discontinuation of pad usage after treatment, while 25.5% continued to use one or more pads. In this group are included 7.2% of patients who had no improvement.

In 60.3% of cases, additional injections were deemed necessary, with a median of 1 (p25–p75: 0–2) additional treatment (Table 1) and a median time until the second injection of 18 months (p25–p75: 11–29).

Table 1. Number of patients by number of treatments requested after the first procedure.

Number of Treatments	Number of Patients (%)
0	146 (39.7)
1	114 (30.9)
2	61 (16.6)
3	24 (6.5)
4	8 (2.2)
5	7 (1.9)
6	6 (1.6)
7	1 (0.3)
8	1 (0.3)

The number of pads used at baseline predicted the chance of being dry after botulinum toxin injection. As a matter of fact, it was observed that the lower the number of pads used before the treatment, the higher the likelihood of achieving a pad-free situation. Specifically, women who discontinued pads after onabotulinumtoxinA (onabotA) had an average of 3.5 pads pre-OnabotA while those who still required pads had an average of 4.8 pads pre-OnabotA ($p < 0.05$). Additionally, patients who had undergone sling placement were less likely to achieve continence. Among those without previous sling placement, 77.9% achieved pad-free status after OnabotA treatment compared with 65.8% among those with prior sling placement ($p < 0.05$). No statistically significant relationship was identified between BMI and the number of pads before and after injection.

Regarding the request for new treatments, women who repeated the injection at least twice were, on average, younger at the time of diagnosis (57.3 years, SD $\pm$ 16.1) compared to those who did not repeat injections (61.7 years, SD $\pm$ 13.1) ($p < 0.05$). Furthermore, patients who reported satisfaction were more likely to undergo repeated treatment than those who expressed dissatisfaction ($p < 0.05$).

In the multivariate analysis model, which included the variables age, BMI, previous slings, and the previous number of pads, only the previous number of pads was an independent predictor of having zero pads after injection (adjusted OR 1.12; $p = 0.042$).

The complications associated with the treatments were mild. There were 4 patients with urinary retention requiring temporary urethral catheterization (1.1%) and 29 (7.9%) with symptoms of urinary tract infection treated with oral antibiotics.

3. Discussion

Only onabotulinumtoxinA (Botox®, Allergan, Inc., Irvine, CA, USA) 100U is licensed in Europe to treat UUI/OAB, and it is relevant to note that it is more effective in curing UUI than antimuscarinics, being a third-line treatment based on the assumption that intervention therapy should follow oral medication [2,3]. Sacral nerve stimulation is also a third-line treatment; however, so far, the trials demonstrated that the neuromodulation is comparable not with 100 U but with 200 U of the same toxin. Additionally, the increasing invasiveness, more serious complications, and higher costs of the two-stage implantation procedure should be mentioned, despite the potential need for just one (two, in fact) intervention [4,5]. However, that is beyond the scope of this paper.

The introduction of intravesical botulinum toxin treatment has been a significant advancement. It began to be used to treat medical conditions by the end of the 1970s, but it was only applied in urology in 1988, being used to treat urinary incontinence a few years later [6]. The first significant studies and clinical applications of botulinum toxin for treating UUI emerged around the early 2000s, and by 2009, substantial evidence supported its efficacy for this condition, leading to broader use in clinical practice. It is a neurotoxic protein produced by *Clostridium botulinum*, with seven subtypes. Subtype A has the longest duration of action, which makes it the most clinically relevant [2,6].

Botulinum toxin subtype A consists of a heavy and a light chain linked by a disulfide bond. When it is injected, it infiltrates the nerve terminals and enters the presynaptic neuron membrane through binding of the heavy chain to the synaptic vesicle protein (SV2). The heavy chain of the toxin exhibits an affinity for polygangliosides located on the surface of neuronal terminals, thereby augmenting the toxin's concentration on the neuronal membrane. This heightened concentration enhances the likelihood of the heavy chain encountering the protein acceptor SV2 predominantly expressed within synaptic vesicles. After toxin endocytosis, acidification within the synaptic vesicles precipitates the elimination of the disulfide bond and the dissociation of the two chains. The light chain protein, which is the true active part, is then linked to the synaptosomal nerve-associated protein 25 (SNAP-25). When the light chain links to SNAP-25, it cleaves it and inactivates it [2,6]. By cleaving SNAP-25, it hinders the proper formation of the SNARE (Soluble NSF Attachment Protein Receptor) complex. As the SNARE complex mediates the binding of neurotransmitters vesicles to the plasma membrane of the nerve terminals, so they can fuse and release acetylcholine (Ach), and, consequently, this prevents Ach exocytosis from the vesicles. Why is this Ach blockage so essential? Because if during the voiding phase it plays a crucial role in bladder contraction to facilitate urine evacuation, during the storage phase, its effect is undesirable since there is no physiological parasympathetic input to the lower urinary tract. However, ACh can be spontaneously released from nerves and non-neuronal structures, including the urothelium and suburothelium, during this phase. This release can activate afferent nerves innervating the bladder, potentially causing urgency and UUI. When the cascade of events due to botulin toxin bladder injection occurs, as Ach is not released, it cannot bind to muscarinic receptors on the bladder detrusor muscle, thereby averting undesired contractions [2,7,8]. Furthermore, adding to this motor/efferent modulation, botulinum toxin reduces the expression of sensory receptors in bladder nerves by hampering their transfer from intracellular vesicles to the neuronal membrane, also modulating the sensory/afferent component of the disease [9].

What sets different commercial forms apart is the molecular weight of the accessory protein that covers the toxin. Xeomin® (Merz Pharmaceuticals GmbH, Frankfurt, Germany), Dysport® (Ipsen Biopharm Ltd., Wrexham, UK), and especially Botox® (Allergan, Inc., Irvine, CA, USA) are the best known. Xeomin® (Merz Pharmaceuticals GmbH, Frankfurt, Germany) has a molecular weight of only 150 kDa, Dysport® (Ipsen Biopharm

Ltd., Wrexham, UK) around 400 kDa, and Botox® (Allergan, Inc., Irvine, CA, USA) 900 kDa. Consequently, posology, the potency per weight of each brand, is unique and not interchangeable [10]. This was the reason behind the FDA introducing the non-proprietary names of incobotulinumtoxinA (incobotA) for Xeomin® (Merz Pharmaceuticals GmbH, Frankfurt, Germany), abobotulinumtoxinA (abobotA) for Dysport® (Ipsen Biopharm Ltd., Wrexham, UK), and, as previously mentioned, onabotulinumtoxinA (onabotA) for Botox® (Allergan, Inc., Irvine, CA, USA) [2].

Despite the dose depending on the chosen toxin brand, the preparation method is similar. It is important to note that during reconstitution, vials should be gently stirred rather than shaken, as vigorous agitation may disrupt the delicate disulfide bond linking the light and heavy chains of the botulinum toxin molecule [10]. Regarding its administration, it requires the injection of a toxin solution into the bladder wall, as the toxin fails to cross the urothelium upon instillation into the bladder. Efforts to facilitate this process have so far yielded limited success or await a definitive validation of efficacy. For patients with OAB undergoing a bladder injection of onabotA, the standard administration implies 20 injections of 0.5 mL each, classically sparing the trigone. However, despite these recommendations regarding the number of injection sites, many clinicians opt for a reduced number of injection points. Non-randomized controlled studies have utilized one or three injection sites, each receiving 1–5 mL of solution, in the posterior bladder wall, or alternatively, three to four injections of 2 mL each at the equatorial line of the bladder, with no apparent compromise in efficacy [11–13]. Investigations into injections in the trigone have been predicated on the premise that this region of the bladder harbors the highest density of sensory fibers. It is hypothesized that a combination of injections in the bladder walls and trigone may yield greater effectiveness than injections confined solely to the bladder walls in cases of OAB [14,15]. More recently, some studies explored further the reduced number of injections and a different location, offering reassurance that fewer injections seem equally effective, and that trigone inclusion could be as, or even more, effective, as targeting the lower bladder could reduce the urinary retention by maintaining upper bladder function [16–18]. The depth of injections, whether intradetrusor or suburothelial, has been the subject of a meta-analysis, which found no discernible differences in efficacy or safety. Large-scale clinical trials have not detected antibody formation following initial administration. However, to mitigate the risk of immunosensitization, a 12-week interval between injection cycles is recommended [9,10].

This treatment has successfully addressed a significant percentage of patients who did not respond to previous interventions, with effects lasting for an average of 6 months, according to pivotal trials [14,19]. The primary complications of intradetrusor injections of botulinum toxin A are urinary tract infections and urinary retention. Patients should be informed that they might require temporary (self-)catheterization. Yet, the treatment offers the advantage of virtually no systemic side effects [20].

As UI prevalence is high and its impact on women's lives is substantial, it is imperative to conduct a comprehensive examination of all facets related to its treatment to ensure the delivery of increasingly efficacious care [21,22]. Notwithstanding this, probably because its efficacy has already been established, recent studies analyzing it are scarce, especially in an idiopathic context and even more specifically in the female population. This scarcity is even more pronounced if we consider it from a patient-reported-outcomes perspective, or with apparently less objective measures such as the number of pads, which may actually be the best surrogates for a patient's quality of life. Furthermore, the latest evaluations available focus on urodynamic parameters. Notably, one of the key urodynamic markers for OAB is detrusor hyperactivity, which is not always necessary for diagnosis.

Therefore, when we say that the primary objective of this study is to assess the efficacy of botulinum toxin, we are addressing something directly applicable to real-life practice: this can inform a patient about the probability of no longer needing to use pads following the treatment. It is remarkable that 74.5% of patients reported a complete discontinuation of pad usage post treatment, but it is essential to acknowledge that this rate includes only those achieving complete dryness, as there were women still employing pads but who experienced significant improvements, leading to great changes in their quality of life. As such, of the remaining 25.5% patients, some exhibited a positive response to Botox; and some, with a negative response in the first treatment, underwent a second treatment to address dosage and technical issues as potential causes of the initial failure.

As the main determinants of efficacy, we identified the number of pads used before treatment and a history of sling placement, both exerting influence on treatment outcomes. The former is inherently predictable, given the association between the severity of UI and treatment challenges. Furthermore, certain patients not responsive to conservative management, due to antimuscarinic intolerance, may signify a more easily treatable condition, correlating with a higher success rate [23]. However, the latter finding deviates from prior reports demonstrating similar efficacy in women with or without a history of previous sling surgery [24]. In the present investigation, there appears to be a trend towards a less favorable clinical outcome in patients with a history of prior sling procedures. Despite timely reassessment for obstruction in patients upon UUI development, one could argue that sling surgery often augments bladder outlet resistance, yielding functional consequences even in cases with low post-void residual and high flow rates. Supporting this contention, urinary NGF, elevated in female rats with bladder outlet obstruction, was similarly elevated in reports of patients after sling placement, comparable to levels previously described in patients with overactive bladder [25]. Moreover, some studies suggest that increased bladder outlet resistance after a sling procedure may significantly contribute to the rise of urinary neurotrophins, promoting the sensitization of bladder primary afferents and inducing de novo urgency in susceptible patients [26]. This finding could prompt a new line of inquiry into whether patients with a sling truly have idiopathic UUI or if the sling itself was the cause. In both cases (high number of pads used before treatment and a history of sling placement), we should be more emphatic explaining to the patient the lower probability of success, as expectations are decisive in the therapeutic process. These will be the most challenging patients, but also the ones more in need for a solution.

Despite an average interval of approximately 6 months, pivotal trials indicate the need for repeat injections with intervals ranging from 3 months to over a year [27,28]. Patients received a second injection after a median duration of 18 months. Although surprisingly long, it is important to note that this interval does not necessarily equate to the duration of therapeutic effect. Over nearly 15 years, various factors contributed to this timeframe, albeit some no longer relevant today. Logistical challenges, including temporary follow-up losses and delayed post-Botox evaluations, contributed to this timeframe, with patients often waiting excessively to consult their urologist. Additionally, some patients were still pleased with the tail effect of the previous toxin injection, which means that, although lacking the full influence from the treatment, they were still satisfied, not seeking a new one. It is also noteworthy that some women opted to defer a second treatment even when the initial one was no longer effective, primarily due to the invasiveness of the procedure, carried out in the operating room under sedation, prompting a desire to avoid it.

This highlights the necessity of finding a novel method of botulinum toxin administration. To date, the administration requires the injection of a toxin solution in the bladder wall since the toxin does not traverse the urothelium if instilled in the bladder [29]. Various facilitators for enhancing the transurothelial passage of the toxin have been explored, including liposomes, the reverse thermal gelation TC-3 hydrogel, low-energy shock waves, and electromotive administration [30–33]. However, botulinum toxin encapsulated in liposomes did not produce results robust enough to pursue its development in OAB. It also failed when mixed in reverse thermal biodegradable hydrogel that increases viscosity at body temperature. Three thousand low-energy shock waves delivered during 10 min to the bladder half-filled with a solution containing 100U onabotA provided short-lasting effects. Electromotive administration has also been investigated without success. Facilitators for the passage of the toxin through the urothelium have so far failed or did not show irrefutable efficacy. The use of the needle in a flexible cystoscope, with a local anesthetic agent such as lidocaine, may also allow to perform an in-office procedure, which is simpler for the patients to repeat [34].

This phenomenon is interconnected with the repetition of the procedure across the years. While age at diagnosis and satisfaction emerged as determinants for procedure repetition, certain patients, even those young and satisfied with the results, opted to postpone it even when already losing efficacy. We attribute it to the aforementioned reasons.

Although older patients of the cohort appeared to request fewer treatments, the issue of age prompts further reflection. While the safety of onabotulinumtoxinA administration in elderly patients has been established, the same is not entirely true for previous treatment lines such as anticholinergics. In fact, the chronic use of anticholinergic drugs is increasingly being challenged due to growing evidence that prolonged exposure may lead to cognitive deterioration, particularly among elderly patients already at risk of dementia [35]. Moreover, a systematic review has shown that botulinum toxin injections are significantly more effective in curing UUI compared to any form of oral medication [36]. Given these considerations, should intravesical botulinum toxin be contemplated or even prioritized before anticholinergics, in an aging population?

Another matter of concern is the loss of efficacy over time. While subjective patient perceptions in clinical practice suggest diminishing efficacy with subsequent injections, our findings did not corroborate this observation. Furthermore, studies indicate a reduction in urgency severity associated with long-term therapeutic effects, aligning with real-world practice observations [37].

The principal limitations of our results stem from the retrospective nature of the study and the heterogeneity of clinical records among urologists, including the absence of standardized questionnaires or bladder diaries, which complicates the objective quantification of patient improvement without introducing biases. There are several points where this could be more evident. First, as the number of pads used is not consistently reported in clinical practice, the magnitude of improvement with the injections is probably higher than indicated. Conversely, complications from the treatment are likely underreported, as some are resolved before patients contact their urologist or are not detailed in clinical records. Additionally, demographics such as BMI, which we did not find to correlate with outcomes, might have shown correlations if we had a larger dataset, as analyses from randomized studies showed that a higher BMI is associated with a decreased time to recurrence [38]. Finally, regarding patient selection, it is possible that relevant information from patient clinical history was not recorded, preventing us from excluding women with identified causes of UUI.

As we acknowledge that many of the limitations of this study are due to its retrospective nature, future research should ideally be conducted prospectively, with all research questions defined in advance. Women for whom the treatment is effective but still decide to discontinue are intriguing. Does the procedural context—typically performed in an operating room—play a significant role? Do they never return to their baseline status and feel good enough? These are questions that remain to be addressed.

4. Conclusions

Intravesical botulinum toxin is a highly effective treatment. A clear correlation exists between a lower pre-procedural pad usage and a higher likelihood of achieving continence. Contrarily, patients with a history of sling placement for stress urinary incontinence who developed UUI exhibited a reduced likelihood of attaining continence. Furthermore, younger women at the time of diagnosis demonstrated an increased inclination to seek repeated injections, a trend mirrored in patients expressing greater satisfaction with the initial procedure. Surprisingly, in real-life conditions, patients often delayed the next injection longer than anticipated.

5. Materials and Methods

This is a retrospective observational cohort study. Women over 18 years old with a diagnosis of UUI, included or not in the OAB syndrome, were included if they were refractory to conservative treatment. All eligible patients had not been adequately managed with one or more anticholinergics and/or b3-adrenergic receptor agonists for UUI treatment, due to insufficient efficacy or intolerable side effects. Patients underwent treatment with botulinum toxin injection between 2010 and 2023. Women with an identified cause for their clinical condition were excluded, as well as those whose first treatment was performed in the last quarter of 2023, as it was deemed insufficient time for a proper reassessment of the need for new injections.

OnabotulinumtoxinA (Botox®, Allergan, Inc., Irvine, CA, USA) was the administered toxin in all patients. It was administered under light sedation using a rigid cystoscope and a 22-gauge needle. The product was injected at 20 sites, with each injection delivering 0.5 mL, distributed throughout the bladder [11]. In recent years, more injections were positioned below the equatorial line. To enhance the distribution area of onabotulinumtoxinA, the bladder was filled with 200 mL of saline. Prophylactic antibiotics were administered concurrently with sedation using a third-generation cephalosporin. Following the procedure, the patient was catheterized, and the catheter was removed a few hours later. However, in recent years, no bladder catheter was left in place post procedure, and the bladder was merely emptied.

Post-operatively, patients were assessed by different doctors, at various time intervals.

The primary outcome was efficacy, evaluated through the cessation of the need for pads. Secondary outcomes included the time between injections, determinants of efficacy, and patient satisfaction assessed through an affirmative response to the question "Are you satisfied?". Variables such as age at diagnosis, BMI, prior suburethral sling placement before UUI diagnosis, the number of pads used before and after the intervention, the number of botulinum toxin treatments, the time between each treatment, and patient satisfaction were assessed. Complications were also measured.

The statistical analysis was conducted using IBM SPSS Statistics version 26.0 (IBM Corp., Armonk, NY, USA). A descriptive analysis of the sample was performed. Frequencies were expressed in percentages, and continuous variables were presented as means and medians, with their respective standard deviation and interquartile range. Student's t-test and chi-square tests were used, considering a p-value < 0.05 as statistically significant. Binary logistic regression was used to evaluate the independent predictive value of the number of pre-injection pads and the previous use of a sling, adjusted for age and BMI, as predictors of the primary outcome.

This study was approved by the ethics committee of the Centro Hospitalar Universitário São João (CES 293/2023).

Author Contributions: Conceptualization, M.M. and F.C.; methodology, F.C.; software, formal analysis, F.B.; investigation, M.M.; data curation, J.D.S. and M.H.; writing—original draft preparation, M.M.; writing—review and editing, M.M., C.S. and F.C.; supervision, F.C. All authors have read and agreed to the published version of the manuscript.

Funding: This research received no external funding.

Institutional Review Board Statement: The study was conducted in accordance with the Declaration of Helsinki and approved by the Ethics Committee of the Centro Hospitalar Universitário São João (CES 293/2023).

Informed Consent Statement: Patient consent was waived due to the retrospective nature of the study, without investigational intervention.

Data Availability Statement: The original contributions presented in the study are included in the article, further inquiries can be directed to the corresponding author.

Conflicts of Interest: The authors declare no conflicts of interest.

References

1. Milsom, I.; Irwin, D.E. A Cross-Sectional, Population-Based, Multinational Study of the Prevalence of Overactive Bladder an Lower Urinary Tract Symptoms: Results from the EPIC Study. *Eur. Urol. Suppl.* **2007**, *6*, 4–9. [CrossRef]
2. Partin, A.W.; Dmochowsky, R.R.; Kavoussi, L.R.; Peters, C.A. *Campbell-Walsh-Wein Urology*, 12th ed.; Elsevier: Philadelphia, PA USA, 2020; pp. 2581–2586, 2592, 2638–2639, 2707–2709.
3. Nambiar, A.K.; Arlandis, S.; Bø, K.; Cobussen-Boekhorst, H.; Costantini, E.; de Heide, M.; Farag, F.; Groen, J.; Karavitakis, M Lapitan, M.C.; et al. European Association of Urology Guidelines on the Diagnosis and Management of Female Non-neurogeni Lower Urinary Tract Symptoms. Part 1: Diagnostics, Overactive Bladder, Stress Urinary Incontinence, and Mixed Urinar Incontinence. *Eur. Urol.* **2022**, *82*, 49–59. [CrossRef]
4. Amundsen, C.L.; Komesu, Y.M.; Chermansky, C.; Gregory, W.T.; Myers, D.L.; Honeycutt, E.F.; Vasavada, S.P.; Nguyen, J.N Wilson, T.S.; Harvie, H.S.; et al. Two-Year Outcomes of Sacral Neuromodulation Versus OnabotulinumtoxinA for Refractor Urgency Urinary Incontinence: A Randomized Trial. *Eur. Urol.* **2018**, *74*, 66–73. [CrossRef] [PubMed]
5. Harvie, H.S.; Amundsen, C.L.; Neuwahl, S.J.; Honeycutt, A.A.; Lukacz, E.S.; Sung, V.W.; Rogers, R.G.; Ellington, D.; Ferrand C.A.; Chermansky, C.J.; et al. Cost-Effectiveness of Sacral Neuromodulation versus OnabotulinumtoxinA for Refractory Urgenc Urinary Incontinence: Results of the ROSETTA Randomized Trial. *J. Urol.* **2020**, *203*, 969–977. [CrossRef]
6. Lin, Y.H.; Chiang, B.J.; Liao, C.H. Mechanism of Action of Botulinum Toxin A in Treatment of Functional Urological Disorder *Toxin* **2020**, *12*, 129. [CrossRef] [PubMed]
7. Cruz, F. Targets for botulinum toxin in the lower urinary tract. *Neurourol. Urodyn.* **2014**, *33*, 31–38. [CrossRef] [PubMed]
8. Dolly, J.O.; Lawrence, G.W. Chapter 3: Molecular basis for the therapeutic effectiveness of botulinum neurotoxin type A. *Neurour Urodyn.* **2014**, *33* (Suppl. S3), S14–S20. [CrossRef]
9. Apostolidis, A.; Jacques, T.S.: Freeman, A.; Kalsi, V.; Popat, R.; Gonzales, G.; Datta, S.N.; Ghazi-Noori, S.; Elneil, S.; Dasgupta, et al. Histological changes in the urothelium and suburothelium of human overactive bladder following intradetrusor injectior of botulinum neurotoxin type A for the treatment of neurogenic or idiopathic detrusor overactivity. *Eur. Urol.* **2008**, *53*, 1245–125 [CrossRef] [PubMed]
10. Brin, M.F.; James, C.; Maltman, J. Botulinum toxin type A products are not interchangeable: A review of the evidence. *Biologi* **2014**, *8*, 227–241. [CrossRef]
11. Nitti, V.W.; Dmochowski, R.; Herschorn, S.; Sand, P.; Thompson, C.; Nardo, C.; Yan, X.; Haag-Molkenteller, C. Onabotulinumto inA for the treatment of patients with overactive bladder and urinary incontinence: Results of a phase 3, randomized, placeb controlled trial. *J. Urol.* **2013**, *189*, 2186–2193. [CrossRef] [PubMed]
12. Avallone, M.A.; Sack, B.S.; El-Arabi, A.; Guralnick, M.L.; O'Connor, R.C. Less is more-A pilot study evaluating one to thre intradetrusor sites for injection of onabotulinumtoxinA for neurogenic and idiopathic detrusor overactivity. *Neurourol. Urody* **2017**, *36*, 1104–1107. [CrossRef] [PubMed]
13. Martínez-Cuenca, E.; Bonillo, M.A.; Morán, E.; Broseta, E.; Arlandis, S. Onabotulinumtoxin re-injection for refractory detrus overactivity using 3-4 injection sites: Results of a pilot study. *Urology* **2020**, *137*, 50–54. [CrossRef] [PubMed]
14. Jo, J.K.; Kim, K.N.; Kim, D.W.; Kim, Y.T.; Kim, J.Y.; Kim, J.Y. The effect of onabotulinumtoxinA according to site of injection patients with overactive bladder: A systematic review and meta-analysis. *World J. Urol.* **2018**, *36*, 305–317. [CrossRef] [PubMe
15. Manecksha, R.P.; Cullen, I.M.; Ahmad, S.; McNeill, G.; Flynn, R.; McDermott, T.E.; Grainger, R.; Thornhill, J.A. Prospectiv randomised controlled trial comparing trigone-sparing versus trigone-including intradetrusor injection of abobotulinumtoxin for refractory idiopathic detrusor overactivity. *Eur. Urol.* **2012**, *61*, 928–935. [CrossRef] [PubMed]
16. DiCarlo-Meacham, A.M.; Dengler, K.L.; Welch, E.K.; Brooks, D.I.; Gruber, D.D.; Osborn, D.J.; Scarlotta, L.; Vaccaro, C.M. Reduce versus standard intradetrusor OnabotulinumtoxinA injections for treatment of overactive bladder. *Neurourol. Urodyn.* **2023**, 4 366–374. [CrossRef] [PubMed]
17. MacDiarmid, S.; Glazier, D.B.; McCrery, R.J.; Kennelly, M.J.; Nelson, M.; Ifantides, K.B.; McCammon, K.A. Efficacy and safety an alternative onabotulinumtoxinA injection paradigm for refractory overactive bladder. *Neurourol. Urodyn.* **2024**, *43*, 31– [CrossRef]
18. Kelsey, E.; Wynn, J.; Holmes, A.; McLeod, K. Anatomical location and number of injection sites of intravesical Onabotulinumt inA for females with refractory idiopathic overactive bladder: A scoping review. *Neurourol. Urodyn.* **2024**, *43*, 553–564. [CrossR [PubMed]
19. Chapple, C.R.; Sievert, K.D.; MacDiarmid, S.; Khullar, V.; Radziszweski, P.; Nardo, C.; Thompson, C.; Zhou, J.; Haag-Molkentell C. OnabotulinomtoxiA 100 U significantly improves all idiopathic overactive bladder symptoms and quality of life in patier with overactive bladder and urinary incontinence: A randomised, double-blind, placebo-controlled trial. *Eur. Urol.* **2013**, 249–256. [CrossRef]
20. Hsieh, P.F.; Chiu, H.C.; Chen, K.C.; Chang, C.H.; Chou, E.C. Botulinum toxin A for the Treatment of Overactive Bladder. *Toxi* **2016**, *8*, 59. [CrossRef] [PubMed]
21. Irwin, D.E.; Kopp, Z.S.; Agatep, B.; Milsom, I.; Abrams, P. Worldwide prevalence estimates of lower urinary tract sympton overactive bladder, urinary incontinence and bladder outlet obstruction. *BJU Int.* **2011**, *108*, 1132–1138. [CrossRef] [PubMed]
22. Manso, M.; Botelho, F.; Bulhões, C.; Cruz, F.; Pacheco-Figueiredo, L. Self-reported urinary incontinence in women is higher wi increased age, lower educational level, lower income, number of comorbidities, and impairment of mental health. Results o large, population-based, national survey in Portugal. *World J. Urol.* **2023**, *41*, 3657–3662. [CrossRef] [PubMed]

23. Cox, L.; Cameron, A.P. OnabotulinumtoxinA for the treatment of overactive bladder. *Res. Rep. Urol.* **2014**, *6*, 79–89. [CrossRef] [PubMed]
24. Miotla, P.; Futyma, K.; Cartwright, R.; Bogusiewicz, M.; Skorupska, K.; Markut-Miotla, E.; Rechberger, T. Effectiveness of botulinum toxin injection in the treatment of de novo OAB symptoms following midurethral sling surgery. *Int. Urogynecol. J.* **2016**, *27*, 393–398. [CrossRef] [PubMed]
25. Chai, T.C.; Richter, H.E.; Moalli, P.; Keay, S.; Biggio, J.; Zong, W.; Curto, T.; Kim, H.Y.; Stoddard, A.M.; Kusek, J.W. Inflammatory and tissue remodeling urinary biomarkers before and after mid urethral sling surgery for stress urinary incontinence. *J. Urol.* **2014**, *191*, 703–709. [CrossRef]
26. Antunes-Lopes, T.; Coelho, A.; Pinto, R.; Barros, S.C.; Cruz, C.; Cruz, F.; Silva, C.M. Urinary Neurotrophin Levels Increase in Women With Stress Urinary Incontinence After a Midurethral Sling Procedure. *Urology* **2017**, *99*, 49–56. [CrossRef]
27. Kalsi, V.; Apostolidis, A.; Gonzales, G.; Elneil, S.; Dasgupta, P.; Fowler, C. Early effect on the overactive bladder symptoms following botulinum neurotoxin type A injections for detrusor overactivity. *Eur. Urol.* **2008**, *54*, 181–187. [CrossRef] [PubMed]
28. Sahai, A.; Dowson, C.; Khan, M.; Dasgupta, P.; GKT Botulinum Study Group. Repeated injections of botulinum toxin-A for idiopathic detrusor overactivity. *Urology* **2010**, *75*, 552–558. [CrossRef]
29. Coelho, A.; Cruz, F.; Cruz, C.D.; Avelino, A. Spread of onabotulinumtoxinA after bladder injection. Experimental study using the distribution of cleaved SNAP-25 as the marker of the toxin action. *Eur. Urol.* **2012**, *61*, 1178–1184. [CrossRef]
30. Chuang, Y.C.; Kuo, H.C. A prospective, multicenter, double-blind, randomized trial of bladder instillation of liposome formulation onabotulinumtoxinA for interstitial cystitis/bladder pain syndrome. *J. Urol.* **2017**, *198*, 376–382. [CrossRef] [PubMed]
31. Rappaport, Y.H.; Zisman, A.; Jeshurun-Gutshtat, M.; Gerassi, T.; Hakim, G.; Vinshtok, Y.; Stav, K. Safety and feasibility of intravesical instillation of botulinum toxin-A in hydrogel-based slow-release delivery system in patients with interstitial cystitis-bladder pain syndrome: A pilot study. *Urology* **2018**, *114*, 60–65. [CrossRef] [PubMed]
32. Nageib, M.; El-Hefnawy, A.S.; Zahran, M.H.; El-Tabey, N.A.; Sheir, K.Z.; Shokeir, A.A. Delivery of intravesical botulinum toxin A using low-energy shockwaves in the treatment of overactive bladder: A preliminary clinical study. *Arab. J. Urol.* **2019**, *17*, 216–220. [CrossRef] [PubMed]
33. Kajbafzadeh, A.M.; Montaser-Kouhsari, L.; Ahmadi, H.; Sotoudeh, M. Intravesical electromotive botulinum toxin type A administration: Part I—Experimental study. *Urology* **2011**, *77*, 1460–1464. [CrossRef] [PubMed]
34. Pereira e Silva, R.; Ponte, C.; Lopes, F.; Palma Dos Reis, J. Alkalinized lidocaine solution as a first-line local anesthesia protocol for intradetrusor injection of onabotulinum toxin A: Results from a double-blinded randomized controlled trial. *Neurourol. Urodyn.* **2020**, *39*, 2471–2479. [CrossRef]
35. Coupland, A.C.; Hill, T.; Dening, T.; Morriss, R.; Moore, M.; Hippisley-Cox, J. Anticholinergic Drug Exposure and the Risk of Dementia: A Nested Case-Control Study. *JAMA Intern. Med.* **2019**, *179*, 1084–1093. [CrossRef] [PubMed]
36. Drake, M.J.; Nitti, V.W.; Ginsberg, D.A.; Brucker, B.M.; Hepp, Z.; McCool, R.; Glanville, J.M.; Fleetwood, K.; James, D.; Chapple, C.R. Comparative assessment of the efficacy of onabotulinumtoxinA and oral therapies (anticholinergics and mirabegron) for overactive bladder: A systematic review and network meta-analysis. *BJU Int.* **2017**, *120*, 611–622. [CrossRef] [PubMed]
37. Kuo, H. Reduction of urgency severity is associated with long-term therapeutic effect after intravesical onabotulinumtoxin A injection for idiopathic detrusor overactivity. *Neurourol. Urodyn.* **2011**, *30*, 1497–1502. [CrossRef] [PubMed]
38. Hendrickson, W.K.; Xie, G.; Rahn, D.D.; Amundsen, C.L.; Hokanson, J.A.; Bradley, M.; Smith, A.L.; Sung, V.W.; Visco, A.G.; Luo, S.; et al. Predicting outcomes after intradetrusor onabotulinumtoxina for non-neurogenic urgency incontinence in women. *Neurourol. Urodyn.* **2022**, *41*, 432–447. [CrossRef]

toxins

MDPI

Systematic Review

Adverse Effects of Intravesical OnabotulinumtoxinA Injection in Patients with Idiopathic Overactive Bladder or Neurogenic Detrusor Overactivity: A Systematic Review and Meta-Analysis of Randomized Controlled Studies

Ping-Hsuan Yu [1,2,3,4] and Chung-Cheng Wang [1,5,*]

1 Department of Urology, En Chu Kong Hospital, College of Medicine, National Taiwan University, New Taipei City 237414, Taiwan; benbenben642001@hotmail.com
2 Department of Urology, Taipei Veterans General Hospital, Taipei 112201, Taiwan
3 Department of Urology, College of Medicine, National Yang Ming Chiao Tung University, Taipei 112304, Taiwan
4 Shu-Tien Urological Science Research Center, National Yang Ming Chiao Tung University, Taipei 112304, Taiwan
5 Department of Biomedical Engineering, Chung Yuan Christian University, Taoyuan 320314, Taiwan
* Correspondence: ericwcc@ms27.hinet.net; Tel.: +886-26723456 (ext. 6620); Fax: +886-26729887

Abstract: Despite the efficacy of onabotulinumtoxinA, its safety profile remains a concern. This meta-analysis reviewed the major adverse events (AEs) associated with intravesical onabotulinumtoxinA treatment in patients with neurogenic detrusor overactivity (NDO) and idiopathic overactive bladder (iOAB). Randomized controlled trials (RCTs) conducted between January 2000 and December 2022 were searched for adult patients administered different onabotulinumtoxinA dosages or onabotulinumtoxinA vs. placebo. Quality assessment was performed using the Cochrane Collaboration tool, and statistical analysis was performed using Review Manager version 5.3. A total of 26 RCTs were included in the analysis, including 8 on NDO and 18 on iOAB. OnabotulinumtoxinA vs. placebo significantly increased the urinary tract infection (UTI) incidence in patients with NDO (relative risk, or RR, 1.54) and iOAB (RR, 2.53). No difference in the RR with different onabotulinumtoxinA dosages was noted. Urinary retention was frequent with onabotulinumtoxinA use in the NDO (RR, 6.56) and iOAB (RR, 7.32) groups. Similar observations were made regarding the risks of de novo clean intermittent catheterization (CIC). The risk of voiding difficulty increased with onabotulinumtoxinA use in patients with iOAB. Systemic AEs of onabotulinumtoxinA, including muscle weakness (RR, 2.79) and nausea (RR, 3.15), were noted in patients with NDO; most systemic AEs had a low incidence and were sporadic.

Keywords: adverse effects; neurogenic detrusor overactivity; idiopathic overactive bladder; onabotulinumtoxinA; meta-analysis

Key Contribution: The risk of urinary tract infection, urinary retention, and de novo clean intermittent catheterization increased after intravesical onabotulinumtoxinA injection in the NDO and iOAB groups but did not vary with increasing dosages. Most AEs were localized to the urinary tract and were controlled well.

1. Introduction

Overactive bladder (OAB) is defined as urinary urgency with or without urgency urinary incontinence, along with other storage symptoms such as daytime frequency and nocturia, without evidence of urinary tract infection (UTI) or other pathological entities [1,2]. Based on the existence of underlying neurological diseases, OAB can be further classified into two different types: neurogenic detrusor overactivity (NDO) and idiopathic overactive bladder (iOAB). NDO generally results from multiple sclerosis (MS) or spinal cord injury (SCI) [3,4]. The prevalence of OAB ranges from 12% to 19%, and it is a common health problem that has a negative impact on many patients physically, mentally, and socially [3,5,6]

Multiple approaches have been applied for the treatment of OAB, ranging from non-pharmacological treatments, such as behavioral modifications and pelvic floor muscle training, to medications, including antimuscarinics and beta-3 adrenoreceptor agonists [7,8]. However, some patients still exhibit refractory symptoms with oral medications, while others may be intolerant to a high rate of adverse effects (AEs), including xerostomia, blurred vision, constipation, cognitive dysfunction, or high blood pressure [9,10]. In such circumstances, intravesical onabotulinumtoxinA injection, posterior tibial nerve stimulation, and sacral neuromodulation are invasive but feasible alternative treatment options [11,12].

OnabotulinumtoxinA, a specific formulation of botulinum toxin A, is a neurotoxin produced by the anaerobic bacterium *Clostridium botulinum* [13]. It inhibits acetylcholine release from presynaptic neurons by binding to synaptic vesicle glycoprotein 2A, thereby paralyzing muscle contraction [14,15]. The use of intravesical onabotulinumtoxinA injection was first reported by Schurch in 2000 in patients with NDO to reduce excessive detrusor spasticity [16]. After injection with onabotulinumtoxinA, the treatment effects can last for at least 6 months [17]. Gradually, onabotulinumtoxinA treatment has been widely accepted for patients with NDO and iOAB. Intravesical onabotulinumtoxinA injections were approved by the Food and Drug Administration in 2011 to treat urinary incontinence associated with NDO. Currently, the American Urological Association and European Association of Urology guidelines recommend intravesical onabotulinumtoxinA injection as a third-line treatment for OAB [18,19].

Although its efficacy and duration of effectiveness are well recognized, the safety profile of onabotulinumtoxinA remains a concern. Intravesical onabotulinumtoxinA injection causes AEs, particularly a substantially high incidence of UTI and urinary retention [20,21]. Injection of onabotulinumtoxinA inevitably increases the post-void residual volume, thereby increasing the risk of urine retention, de novo clean intermittent catheterization (CIC), and UTI [22]. In addition to AEs localized to the urinary tract, other systemic AEs such as muscle weakness, fatigue, and autonomic dysreflexia have been occasionally reported [23,24].

In this study, we primarily focused on the major AEs associated with intravesical onabotulinumtoxinA treatment, including localized and systemic AEs, in patients with NDO or iOAB. The incidence of each AE under onabotulinumtoxinA injection was recorded, and the increasing risk between different dosages and placebo treatment was evaluated using a meta-analysis.

2. Results

2.1. Study Selection, Characteristics, and Risk of Bias

This review was performed in accordance with the Preferred Reporting Items for Systematic Reviews and Meta-Analyses (PRISMA) guidelines. Initially, 1526 literature sources were identified, and 260 were eliminated owing to duplication. After screening the titles and abstracts, 1185 articles were excluded, leaving only 81 articles for full-text reading. Finally, 26 articles were included in this meta-analysis (Figure 1) [23–43].

This review encompassed 26 literature sources pertaining to randomized controlled trials (RCTs) on bladder onabotulinumtoxinA injections (Table 1). These studies involved 3876 patients diagnosed with NDO or iOAB. Eighteen RCTs, comprising 2904 patients, were related to iOAB (1113 in the placebo group and 1640 in the onabotulinumtoxinA group, with the 151 in the solifenacin group not being analyzed), whereas eight RCTs, including 972 patients, were related to NDO (379 in the placebo group and 593 in the onabotulinumtoxinA group). The etiologies of NDO included MS (n = 550) and SCI (n = 422).

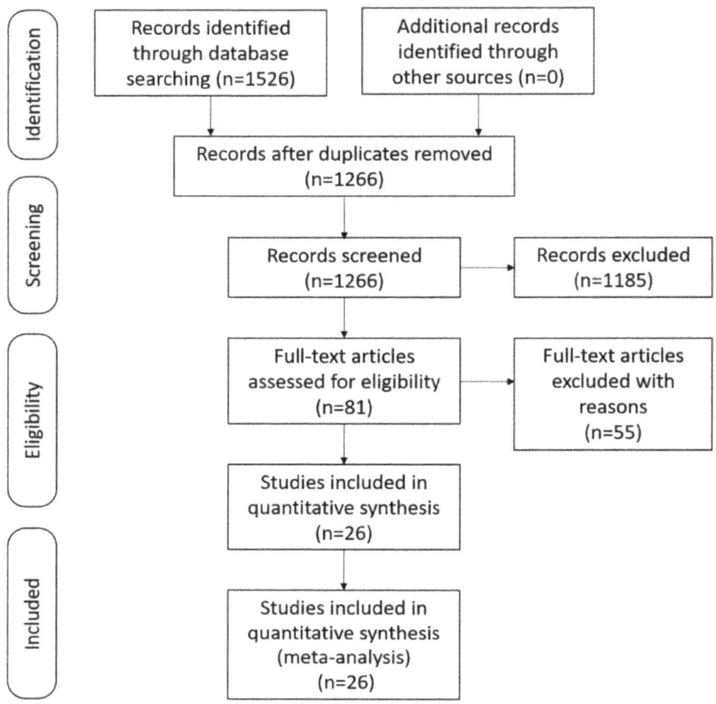

Figure 1. Flow diagram of the study participant selection process.

In the OAB literature, the studies by Dmochowski et al. [35] and Rovner et al. [38] were related to the same cohort in a phase II dose-ranging trial. Since most AEs were detailed in the study by Dmochowski et al., we listed all the literature in Table 1 but only performed an analysis of the study by Dmochowski et al. In addition, Chapple et al. [41] and Nitti et al. [42] studied two cohorts from the EMBARK study group, and Sievert et al. [44] presented the combined data from these two cohorts. We listed the three literature sources; however, most of the analyses focused on the first two articles. Similar conditions existed in the NDO literature, with the studies by Cruz et al. [23], Ginsberg et al. [24], Ginsberg et al. [27], and Rovner et al. [28] all related to the DIGNITY study. This analysis was primarily carried out on the studies by Cruz et al. [23] and Ginsberg et al. [24]. The OAB study by Herschorn et al. [46] included onabotulinumtoxinA, solifenacin, and placebo treatment arms. Our analysis compared the onabotulinumtoxinA arm with a placebo.

Regarding the dose of onabotulinumtoxinA, the onabotulinumtoxinA units in the iOAB trials ranged from 50 U to 300 U, with 100 U being the most commonly administered dose, followed by 200 U. In the NDO trials, most doses were between 200 U and 300 U, except for one RCT in which 100 U botulinum toxin was injected into patients with MS [29]. The AEs have been monitored at different time points in various studies. The incidence of AEs analyzed in this study was mainly focused on the first 24 weeks after the injection.

The risk of bias in all the studies was assessed by two reviewers using the Cochrane Collaboration tool. Table 2 presents the results of the studies.

Table 1. Characteristics of the individual studies.

First Author	Year	Region	No. of Patients (Female)	Ages, Means (SD)	Design	Classification	Basic Diseases	Randomization	AEs Follow-Up (Weeks)
Schurch [25]	2005	Switzerland, Belgium, and France	59 (23)	41	RCT	NDO	MS6, SCI53	BTX 200U 19, BTX 300U 19, Placebo 21	2, 6, 12, 18, 24
Herschorn [26]	2011	Canada	57 (23)	42.8	RCT	NDO	MS19, SCI38	BTX 300U 28, Placebo 29	6, 24, 36
Cruz [23]	2011	Europe, North America, Latin America, South Africa, and Asia Pacific	275 (155)	46 (13.1), 44.4 (13.9), 46.9 (13.4)	RCT	NDO	MS154, SCI121	BTX 200U 92, BTX 300U 91, Placebo 92	At least 12
Ginsberg [24]	2012	USA and Europe	416 (245)	46 (13)	RCT	NDO	MS227, SCI189	BTX 200U 135, BTX 300U 132, Placebo 149	At least 12
Ginsberg [27]	2013	Europe, North America, Latin America, South Africa, and Asia Pacific	691 (400)	45.9	RCT	NDO	MS381, SCI310	BTX 200U 227, BTX 300U 223, Placebo 241	At least 12
Rovner [28]	2013	Europe, North America, Latin America, South Africa, and Asia Pacific	691 (400)	45.9 (13.3), 45.6 (13.0), 46.2 (13.3)	RCT	NDO	MS381, SCI310	BTX 200U 227, BTX 300U 223, Placebo 241	At least 12
Tullman [29]	2018	Europe, North America	144 (127)	51.6 (10.3)	RCT	NDO	MS144	BTX 100U 66, Placebo 78	2, 6, 12
Honda [30]	2021	Japan	21 (4)	50.9 (14.1), 47.2 (18.3)	RCT	NDO	SCI21	BTX 200U 11, Placebo 10	At least 12
Sahai [31]	2007	UK	34 (19)	49.8, 50.8	RCT	iOAB	NA	BTX 200U 16, Placebo 18	4, 12, 24
Brubaker [32]	2008	USA	43 (43)	64.7 (14.5), 69.2 (13.5)	RCT	iOAB	NA	BTX 200U 28, Placebo 15	Within 52
Cohen [33]	2009	USA	44	NA	RCT	iOAB	NA	BTX 150U 22, BTX 100U 22	2, 6, 12, 24
Flynn [34]	2009	USA	22	66	RCT	iOAB	NA	BTX 200U or 300U 15, Placebo 7	3, 6

Table 1. *Cont.*

First Author	Year	Region	No. of Patients (Female)	Ages, Means (SD)	Design	Classification	Basic Diseases	Randomization	AEs Follow-Up (Weeks)
Dmochowski [35]	2010	North America, Europe	313 (288)	58.8	RCT	iOAB	NA	BTX 50U 57, BTX 100U 54, BTX 150U 49, BTX 200U 53, BTX 300U 56, Placebo 44	2, 6, 12, 18, 24, 30, 36
Altaweel [36]	2011	Saudi Arabia	22	NA	RCT	iOAB	NA	BTX 100U 11, BTX 200U 11	2, 12
Dowson [37]	2011	UK	23	NA	RCT	iOAB	NA	BTX 100U 10, Placebo 13	4, 12
Rovner [38]	2011	North America, Europe	313 (288)	58.8	RCT	iOAB	NA	BTX 50U 57, BTX 100U 54, BTX 150U 49, BTX 200U 53, BTX 300U 56, Placebo 44	2, 6, 12, 18, 24, 30, 36
Denys [39]	2012	France	99 (87)	61.6 (14.0)	RCT	iOAB	NA	BTX 50U 23, BTX 100U 23, BTX 150U 30, Placebo 31	4, 12, 20, 24
Tincello [40]	2012	UK	240 (240)	60.7, 58.2	RCT	iOAB	NA	BTX 200U 122, Placebo 118	6, 12, 24
Chapple [41]	2013	USA and Europe	548 (473)	59.5 (15.5), 59.2 (14.1)	RCT	iOAB	NA	BTX 100U 277, Placebo 271	Within 24
Nitti [42]	2013	USA, Canada	557 (497)	61.7 (12.7), 61 (13.1)	RCT	iOAB	NA	BTX 100U 280, Placebo 277	Within 24
Jabs [43]	2013	Canada	21 (21)	63 (9.4), 63.8 (11.2)	RCT	iOAB	NA	BTX 100U 11, Placebo 10	6, 12, 24
Sievert [44]	2014	Europe, North America	1105 (970)	60.6 (14.2), 60.1 (13.6)	RCT	iOAB	NA	BTX 100U 557, Placebo 548	Within 24

Table 1. *Cont.*

First Author	Year	Region	No. of Patients (Female)	Ages, Means (SD)	Design	Classification	Basic Diseases	Randomization	AEs Follow-Up (Weeks)
Abdelwahab [45]	2015	Egypt	80 (63)	30.22 (8.37), 31.35 (7.61)	RCT	iOAB	NA	BTX 100U 40, BTX 200U 40	4, 12, 24, 36
Herschorn [46]	2017	North America, Europe	356 (308)	62.0 (12.3)	RCT	iOAB	NA	BTX 100U 145, Solifenacin 151, Placebo 60	2, 6, 12, 18, 24
Yokoyama [47]	2020	Japan	248 (186)	65.6 (12.4), 66.2 (12.2)	RCT	iOAB	NA	BTX 100U 124, Placebo 124	12
McCammon [48]	2021	USA	254 (226)	60.8 (12.4)	RCT	iOAB	NA	BTX 100U 129, Placebo 125	12

AE: adverse effect; BTX: onabotulinumtoxinA; iOAB: idiopathic overactive bladder; MS: multiple sclerosis; NA: not applicable; NDO: neurogenic detrusor overactivity; RCT: randomized controlled trial; SCI: spinal cord injury; SD: standard deviation.

Table 2. Risks of bias in the individual studies.

First Author	Year	Random Sequence Generation (Selection Bias)	Allocation Concealment (Selection Bias)	Blinding of Participants and Personnel (Performance Bias)	Blinding of Outcome Assessment (Detection Bias)	Incomplete Outcome Data (Attrition Bias)	Selective Reporting (Reporting Bias)	Other Bias
Schurch	2005	Low	Low	Low	Low	Low	Low	Unclear
Herschorn	2011	Low	Low	Low	Low	Low	Low	Unclear
Cruz	2011	Low	Low	Low	Low	Low	Low	Unclear
Ginsberg	2012	Low	Low	Low	Low	Low	Low	Unclear
Ginsberg	2013	Low	Low	Low	Low	Low	Low	Unclear
Rovner	2013	Low	Low	Low	Low	Low	Low	Unclear
Tullman	2018	Low	Low	Low	Low	Low	Low	Unclear
Honda	2021	Low	Unclear	Low	Low	Low	Low	Unclear
Sahai	2007	Low	Low	Low	Low	Unclear	Low	Unclear
Brubaker	2008	Unclear	Unclear	Low	Unclear	Low	Low	Unclear
Cohen	2009	Low	Low	Low	Unclear	Low	Low	Unclear
Flynn	2009	Low	Low	Low	Unclear	Low	Low	Unclear
Dmochowski	2010	Low	Unclear	Low	Low	Low	Low	Unclear
Altaweel	2011	Low	Low	Low	Low	Low	Low	Unclear
Dowson	2011	Low	Low	Low	Low	Unclear	Low	Unclear
Rovner	2011	Low	Low	Unclear	Low	Low	Low	Unclear
Denys	2012	Low	Unclear	Low	Low	Low	Low	Unclear
Tincello	2012	Low	Low	Low	Low	Low	Low	Unclear
Chapple	2013	Low	Low	Low	Unclear	Low	Low	Unclear
Nitti	2013	Low	Low	Unclear	Low	Low	Low	Unclear
Jabs	2013	Unclear	Low	Low	Low	Low	Low	Unclear
Sievert	2014	Unclear	Low	Low	Unclear	Low	Low	Unclear
Abdelwahab	2015	Low	Unclear	Low	Unclear	Low	Low	Unclear
Herschorn	2017	Unclear	Unclear	Low	Low	Low	Low	Unclear
Yokoyama	2020	Unclear	Low	Low	Low	Low	Low	Unclear
McCammon	2021	Low	Low	Low	Low	Low	Low	Unclear

2.2. Adverse Effects Localized to Urinary Tract

In all the articles, most AEs were localized to the urinary tract, with minimal or no systemic effects. In addition, most AEs were transient and reversible. UTI, urinary retention, and voiding difficulties were the most prevalent AEs.

2.2.1. Urinary Tract Infections

UTI was the most frequently mentioned AE in all the studies. The definition of UTI varied among the studies. The most common definition was bacteriuria, along with more than five white blood cells in the high-power field. Some studies defined UTI based solely on urine strip tests or urine cultures, whereas others did not provide a clear definition.

All eight articles involving patients with NDO reported the incidence of UTI. At baseline, the pooled UTI rate in the NDO placebo group was higher than that in the iOAB placebo group (29.2% vs. 9.4%). With increased treatment dosages for NDO, the pooled incidence of UTI in the onabotulinumtoxinA group was 48.4% (relative risk [RR], 1.54; confidence interval [CI], 1.30–1.83; $p < 0.00001$) (Figure 2). The RRs for the 200 U vs. placebo and 300 U vs. placebo groups were similar (1.47 and 1.46). Consequently, no significant difference in the incidence of UTI was observed between the 300 U and 200 U groups (RR, 1.06; CI, 0.89–1.26; $p = 0.51$) (Figure S1a).

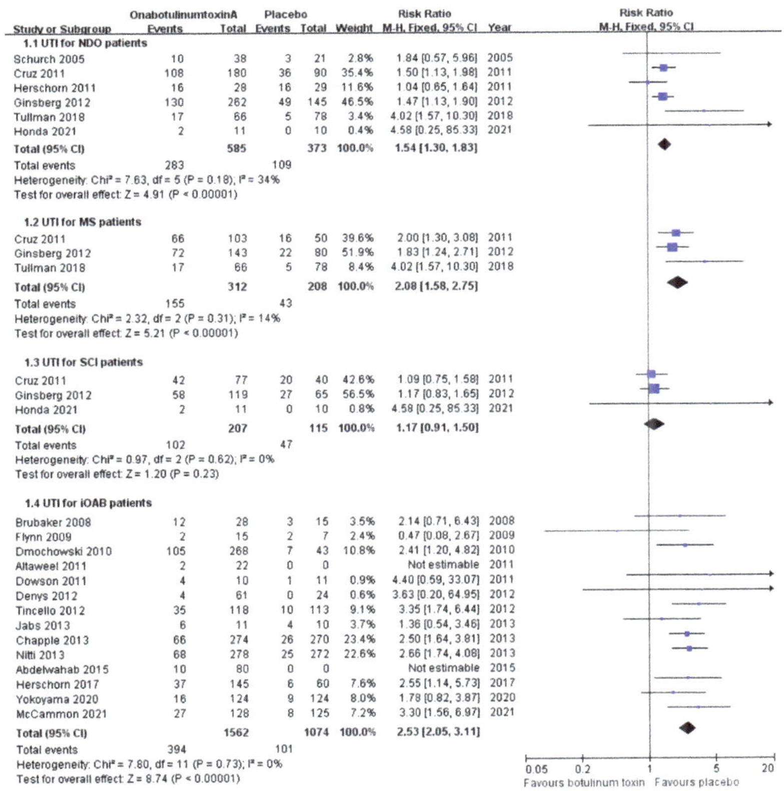

Figure 2. Forest plots of the incidence of urinary tract infection in patients with neurogenic detrusor overactivity due to all causes, multiple sclerosis, spinal cord injury, and idiopathic overactive bladder. iOAB: idiopathic overactive bladder; MS: multiple sclerosis; NDO: neurogenic detrusor overactivity; SCI: spinal cord injury; UTI: urinary tract infection.

When comparing the two etiologies of NDO, most patients with SCI had already regularly undergone CIC. Therefore, we analyzed the incidence of UTI among the two etiologies separately. The RR of the incidence of UTI in patients with MS treated with onabotulinumtoxinA was 2.08 (CI, 1.58–2.75; $p < 0.00001$), which was higher than the RR of all the patients with NDO and patients with SCI (Figure 2). The incidence of UTI between the 300 U and 200 U dosages in patients with MS showed no significant difference (RR, 1.10; CI, 0.88–1.37; $p = 0.40$) (Figure S1b). On the contrary, in patients with SCI, no difference in risk between the onabotulinumtoxinA and placebo groups was observed (RR, 1.17; CI, 0.91–1.50; $p = 0.23$) (Figure 2).

Regarding the patients with iOAB, we analyzed 14 studies that evaluated the UTI incidence following onabotulinumtoxinA treatment. The incidence of UTI between the combined onabotulinumtoxinA and placebo groups showed a significant difference (RR, 2.53; CI, 2.05–3.11; $p < 0.00001$) (Figure 2). The incidence of UTI in the onabotulinumtoxinA 100 U group was 22.7%, compared with 9.4% in the placebo group. The incidence of UTI in the onabotulinumtoxinA 200 U group was 32.1%. Although a dose-dependent rising trend was observed, the RR when comparing 200 U to 100 U did not reach a significant difference (RR, 1.44; CI, 0.94–2.20; $p = 0.09$) (Figure S1c).

Acute pyelonephritis (APN) is a relatively severe AE that can develop even after treatment. APN was mentioned in two studies on iOAB and three studies on NDO, and it appeared to be more sporadic than drug-related APN. One patient in the onabotulinumtoxinA 100 U group and another patient in the 50 U group experienced APN after treatment for iOAB. Three patients in the placebo group for NDO and one patient in the 300 U group were diagnosed with APN after treatment.

Urosepsis is worth noting because of its potentially lethal nature. This issue was addressed in two main studies on NDO [23,24], and it appeared to be more related to the invasive procedure than to onabotulinumtoxinA. Two patients in the placebo group experienced urosepsis, with an incidence of 0.9%.

2.2.2. Urinary Retention

Urinary retention was another major AE commonly reported after treatment with onabotulinumtoxinA. In some studies, urinary retention was defined as a post-void residual volume of >200 mL requiring CIC. However, some studies have defined urinary retention based solely on clinical judgment. The proportion of male patients in each study may have led to distinct results.

Regarding NDO, two articles related to the DIGNITY study [23,24], Tullman et al. [29] and Honda et al. [30], investigated the incidence of urinary retention. The incidence of urinary retention was 20.4% in the onabotulinumtoxinA group, compared with 2.8% in the placebo group (RR, 6.56; CI, 3.43–12.54; $p < 0.00001$) (Figure 3). It is likely that many patients with SCI already underwent CIC (84.8% of patients with SCI underwent CIC at baseline, according to the data of the DIGNITY study [23,24,27,28]). Therefore, the evaluation of urinary retention in this patient group was not straightforward.

By focusing only on patients with MS, the RR could reach 7.82 (CI, 3.71–16.49; $p < 0.00001$) (Figure 3). The combined incidence of urinary retention in patients with SCI was 1.7%, 7.4%, and 4.0% in the placebo, 200 U, and 300 U groups, respectively, whereas the combined incidence of urinary retention in patients with MS was 3.4%, 15.2%, 29.5%, and 39.3% in the placebo, 100 U, 200 U, and 300 U groups, respectively. Although a dose-dependent increasing trend in risk was observed, there was no significant difference between the 200 U and 300 U treatments in all the patients with NDO or the MS-only patients (Figures S2a and S3a).

Although most patients with SCI already undergo regular CIC, the incidence of de novo CIC in patients with SCI who are yet to undergo CIC and in patients with MS remains a concern in terms of higher onabotulinumtoxinA injection doses. For all the patients with NDO without a history of CIC, the risk of de novo CIC for all causes was 2.61 times higher than that for the placebo group; for the MS-only patients, the risk was 2.92 times higher than that for the placebo group (Figure 3). However, the difference in the treatment dose did not affect the risk in all the patients with NDO or the patients with only MS (Figures S2b and S3b).

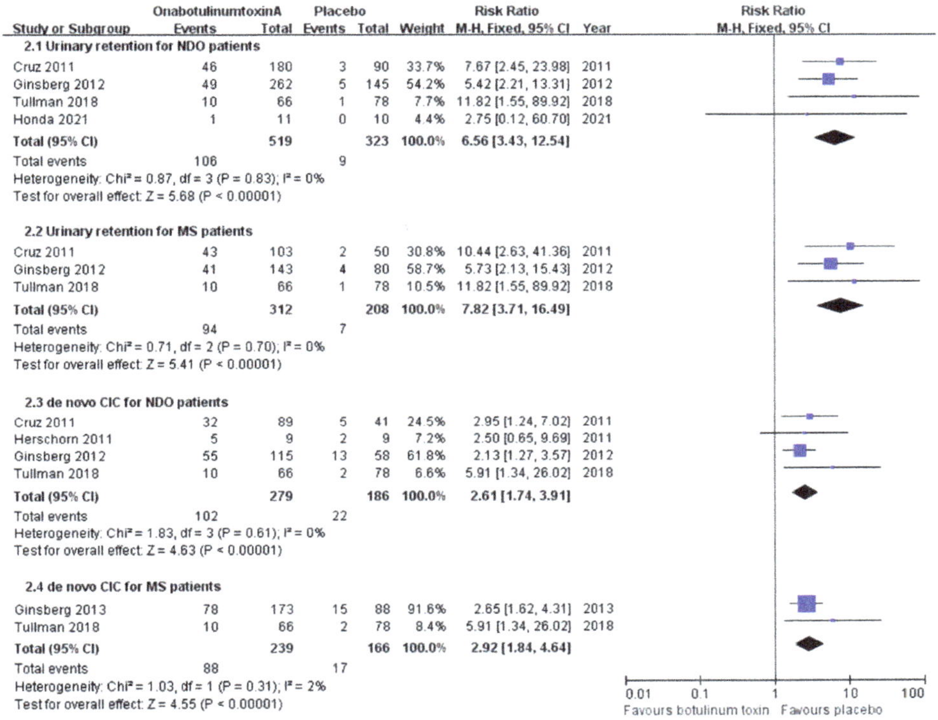

Figure 3. Forest plots of the incidence of urinary retention and de novo clean intermittent catheterization in patients with neurogenic detrusor overactivity due to all causes and neurogenic detrusor overactivity due to multiple sclerosis. CIC: clean intermittent catheterization; MS: multiple sclerosis; NDO: neurogenic detrusor overactivity.

Regarding iOAB, ten studies addressed urinary retention. Accordingly, the pooled retention rates were approximately 1.0% in the placebo group, 6.7% in the onabotulinumtoxinA 100 U group, and 20.1% in the onabotulinumtoxinA 200 U group. The risk of urinary retention for all the onabotulinumtoxinA doses was 7.32 times higher than that for the placebo group (CI, 3.95–13.58; $p < 0.00001$) (Figure 4). When comparing 200 U to 100 U, the increased risk of urinary retention was not significant (RR, 1.34; CI, 0.66–2.72; $p = 0.42$) (Figure S4a). Several studies including patients with iOAB have objectively evaluated the volume of residual urine before and after treatment. Using a cutoff value of 200 mL for residual urine, only 0.3% of patients in the placebo group had residual urine exceeding 200 mL after treatment. After treatment with onabotulinumtoxinA, the incidence of residual urine exceeding 200 mL was 9.6% (10.09 times the risk; CI, 3.80–26.81; $p < 0.00001$).

Study or Subgroup	OnabotulinumtoxinA Events	OnabotulinumtoxinA Total	Placebo Events	Placebo Total	Weight	Risk Ratio M-H, Fixed, 95% CI	Year
3.1 Urinary retention for iOAB patients							
Brubaker 2008	12	28	0	15	5.1%	13.79 [0.87, 217.93]	2008
Cohen 2009	2	44	0	0		Not estimable	2009
Dmochowski 2010	55	268	1	43	13.6%	8.82 [1.25, 62.11]	2010
Altaweel 2011	3	22	0	0		Not estimable	2011
Tincello 2012	16	118	5	113	40.2%	3.06 [1.16, 8.09]	2012
Nitti 2013	16	278	1	272	8.0%	15.65 [2.09, 117.23]	2013
Chapple 2013	16	274	1	270	7.9%	15.77 [2.11, 118.06]	2013
Herschorn 2017	10	145	0	60	5.6%	8.77 [0.52, 147.38]	2017
Yokoyama 2020	7	124	2	124	15.7%	3.50 [0.74, 16.52]	2020
McCammon 2021	8	128	0	125	4.0%	16.60 [0.97, 284.65]	2021
Total (95% CI)		**1429**		**1022**	**100.0%**	**7.32 [3.95, 13.58]**	
Total events	145		10				
Heterogeneity: Chi² = 5.64, df = 7 (P = 0.58); I² = 0%							
Test for overall effect: Z = 6.32 (P < 0.00001)							
3.2 CIC for iOAB patients							
Sahai 2007	6	16	0	18	3.1%	14.53 [0.88, 239.18]	2007
Brubaker 2008	12	28	0	15	4.2%	13.79 [0.87, 217.93]	2008
Cohen 2009	2	44	0	0		Not estimable	2009
Flynn 2009	1	15	0	7	4.3%	1.50 [0.07, 32.84]	2009
Dmochowski 2010	39	268	0	43	5.6%	12.92 [0.81, 206.43]	2010
Dowson 2011	3	10	0	11	3.1%	7.64 [0.44, 131.75]	2011
Denys 2012	8	70	1	29	9.2%	3.31 [0.43, 25.32]	2012
Tincello 2012	16	118	5	113	33.2%	3.06 [1.16, 8.09]	2012
Chapple 2013	19	274	2	270	13.1%	9.36 [2.20, 39.80]	2013
Jabs 2013	1	11	0	10	3.4%	2.75 [0.12, 60.70]	2013
Nitti 2013	17	278	0	272	3.3%	34.25 [2.07, 566.67]	2013
Herschorn 2017	9	145	0	60	4.6%	7.94 [0.47, 134.26]	2017
Yokoyama 2020	7	124	2	124	13.0%	3.50 [0.74, 16.52]	2020
Total (95% CI)		**1401**		**972**	**100.0%**	**6.63 [3.80, 11.57]**	
Total events	140		10				
Heterogeneity: Chi² = 7.08, df = 11 (P = 0.79); I² = 0%							
Test for overall effect: Z = 6.66 (P < 0.00001)							

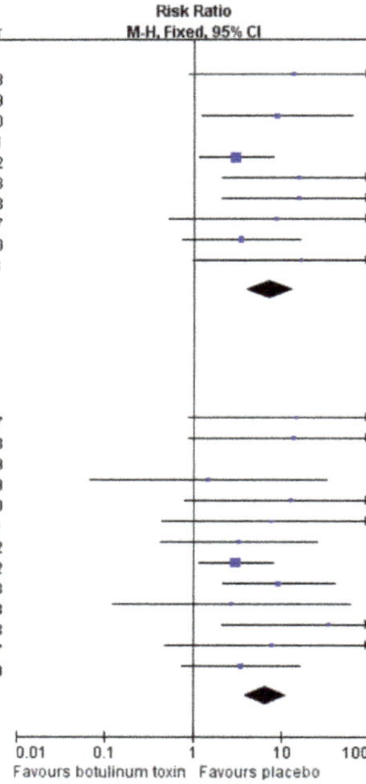

Figure 4. Forest plots of the incidence of urinary retention and clean intermittent catheterization in patients with idiopathic overactive bladder. CIC: clean intermittent catheterization; iOAB: idiopathic overactive bladder.

We also evaluated the possibility of de novo CIC in patients with iOAB. The combined de novo CIC rate in the placebo group was 1.0%. With 100 U onabotulinumtoxinA treatment, the incidence of de novo CIC increased to 6.8% and further increased to 21.0% with 200 U onabotulinumtoxinA treatment. The risk of de novo CIC with onabotulinumtoxinA treatment was 6.63 times higher than that with placebo (CI, 3.80–11.57; $p < 0.00001$) (Figure 4). Dmochowski et al. [35] compared the incidence of de novo CIC between the 200 U onabotulinumtoxinA and 100 U onabotulinumtoxinA groups. The RR was 1.94 with a CI of 0.77–4.86, which still lacked significance (Figure S4b).

2.2.3. Voiding Difficulty

Although not as severe as urinary retention, difficulty in voiding caused inconvenience to patients undergoing onabotulinumtoxinA treatment. Four articles on NDO reported the incidence of voiding difficulty after onabotulinumtoxinA injection. The risk of voiding difficulty with onabotulinumtoxinA injection did not significantly increase, possibly because many patients underwent regular CIC (Figure 5). Eight iOAB studies addressed this issue. The combined incidence of voiding difficulties was approximately 5.3% in the placebo group, including patients with iOAB. The incidence increased to 8.8% in the 100 U group and 21.9% in the 200 U group. We observed not only an increased risk within the combined onabotulinumtoxinA group compared with the placebo group (RR, 1.82; CI, 1.32–2.52; $p = 0.0003$) but also within the 200 U group compared with the 100 U group (RR, 2.25; CI, 1.08–4.71; $p = 0.03$) (Figures 5 and S5).

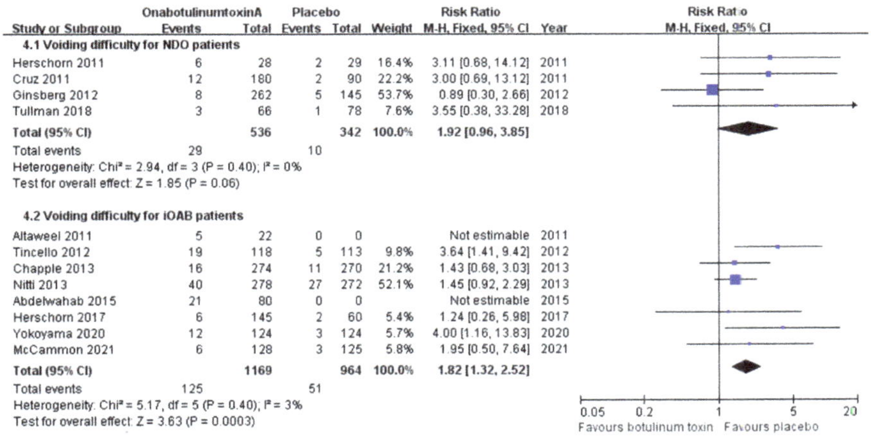

Figure 5. Forest plots of the incidence of voiding difficulty in patients with neurogenic detrusor overactivity and idiopathic overactive bladder. iOAB: idiopathic overactive bladder; NDO: neurogenic detrusor overactivity.

2.2.4. Hematuria

Hematuria was another potential AE. Generally, the risk of hematuria did not increase with onabotulinumtoxinA treatment in patients with NDO or iOAB (Figure S6). Eight articles on iOAB and six articles on NDO discussed this AE. In the iOAB studies, the combined incidence of hematuria was approximately 3.4% in the placebo group and 4.3% in the 100 U group. In the patients with NDO, the combined incidence of hematuria was approximately 4.3% for the placebo group, 5.5% for the 200 U group, and 6.8% in the 300 U group.

2.2.5. Bladder Pain

Despite the fact that an increasing trend of bladder pain was observed with onabotulinumtoxinA injection in patients with NDO, the incidence of bladder pain in the onabotulinumtoxinA group was not significantly higher than that in the placebo group (RR, 2.72; CI, 0.94–7.87; $p = 0.07$) (Figure S6). Four NDO articles reported the incidence of bladder pain. The pooled incidences were 0.9% in the placebo group, 1.2% in the 200 U group, and 5.1% in the 300 U group.

2.3. *Systemic Adverse Effects*

The incidence of systemic AEs was generally low and these AEs usually manifested sporadically. The following were some of the most prevalent systemic AEs.

2.3.1. Muscle Weakness

Because of the muscle-relaxing effects of onabotulinumtoxinA, there are concerns about its systemic effects and the potential for muscle weakness in the extremities. Four studies on NDO and two on iOAB addressed this AE. For the patients with NDO, the combined incidences of muscle weakness were 1.8% in the placebo group, 4.6% in the 200 U group, and 6.6% in the 300 U group. The risk in the onabotulinumtoxinA group was 2.79 times higher than that in the placebo group (CI, 1.18–6.62; $p = 0.02$) (Figure 6). In the iOAB studies, the incidence of muscle weakness was generally low across the different treatment dosages. It was 0.8% in the placebo group and 0.7% in the 200 U group (Figure 6).

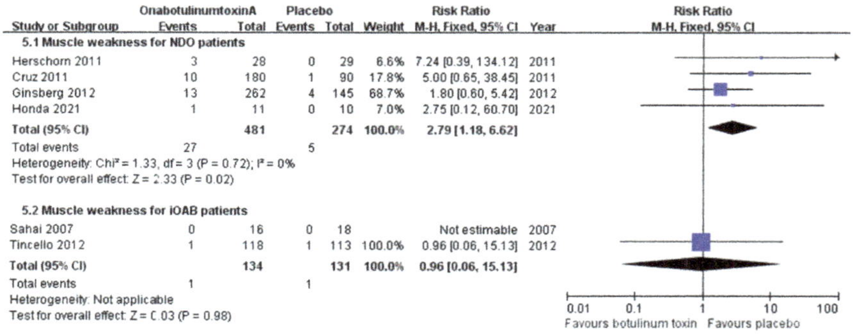

Figure 6. Forest plots of the incidence of muscle weakness in patients with neurogenic detrusor overactivity and idiopathic overactive bladder. iOAB: idiopathic overactive bladder; NDO: neurogenic detrusor overactivity.

2.3.2. Fatigue

The articles from the DIGNITY study [23,24,27,28] evaluated the fatigue rate after injection in patients with NDO. The incidence of fatigue was higher in the patients with MS than in those with SCI who were treated with onabotulinumtoxinA (200 U: 11.6% vs. 1.0%, $p = 0.001$; 300 U: 6.0% vs. 0%, $p = 0.016$). The combined incidences of fatigue were 3.0% in the placebo group, 7.1% in the 200 U group, and 3.2% in the 300 U group. No difference in risk was observed between the onabotulinumtoxinA and placebo groups (Figure S7).

2.3.3. Symptoms Related to the Digestive System (Nausea, Diarrhea, and Constipation)

AEs related to digestive symptoms, including nausea, diarrhea, and constipation, were reported in numerous NDO studies. The risk of diarrhea and constipation did not increase with onabotulinumtoxinA injection (diarrhea: RR, 1.11; CI, 0.59–2.09; $p = 0.75$, constipation: RR, 1.67; CI, 0.72–3.86; $p = 0.23$). However, the risk of nausea significantly increased with onabotulinumtoxinA injection (RR, 3.15; CI, 1.27–7.81; $p = 0.01$). The combined incidences of nausea were 1.9% in the placebo group, 4.0% in the 200 U group, and 7.0% in the 300 U group (Figure S7).

2.3.4. Pyrexia

The articles from the DIGNITY study [23,24], Schurch et al. [25], and Honda et al. [30] evaluated the incidence of pyrexia. Among the patients with NDO, the pooled risk of pyrexia after treatment was 3.0% in the placebo group, 6.6% in the 200 U group, and 2.6% in the 300 U group. This incidence appeared to be unrelated to the treatment dosage (Figure S7).

2.3.5. Autonomic Dysreflexia

With an increasing possibility of urinary retention, the risk of autonomic dysreflexia may also increase after onabotulinumtoxinA treatment, especially in patients with SCI. Four NDO articles were used to evaluate the risk. The pooled incidence of autonomic dysreflexia was 0.4% in the placebo group. When treated with 200 U onabotulinumtoxinA, the risk increased to 2.0%. In the 300 U group, the risk was 1.7%. The RR of autonomic dysreflexia did not increase significantly when comparing onabotulinumtoxinA treatment with placebo (Figure S7).

3. Discussion

Patients with NDO and iOAB have frequent urinary incontinence and other storage symptoms, which significantly reduce their quality of life [8,9,22]. Behavioral therapy, biofeedback, pharmacotherapy, electrical stimulation, onabotulinumtoxinA injection, and surgical intervention have been considered as effective modalities [7,8,49]. The pharmacotherapeutic agents for NDO and iOAB include muscarinic receptor antagonists and beta-3 agonists such as solifenacin, tolterodine, oxybutynin, and mirabegron. Nevertheless, a certain proportion of patients may complain of suboptimal efficacy or may not tolerate the related AEs [50–52]. Thus, researchers continue to search for other therapeutic options that provide long-term treatment efficacy with few AEs. In recent decades, intravesical onabotulinumtoxinA injections have been widely administered to patients with NDO and iOAB. While the application of onabotulinumtoxinA injection improves urinary symptoms and quality of life, onabotulinumtoxinA injection itself has corresponding AEs [20,53].

In this meta-analysis, we focused on the AEs related to intravesical onabotulinumtoxinA injections in patients with either iOAB or NDO in various RCTs. The AEs were mainly limited to the urinary system and were well tolerated. In the urinary system, the incidence of UTI, urinary retention, and de novo CIC induced by onabotulinumtoxinA treatment was higher than that by placebo in the patients with NDO and iOAB; however, the risk of each AE did not vary with an increase in dosage. An increasing incidence of voiding difficulty was observed solely in the patients with iOAB and tended to increase with increasing dosages. The risks of hematuria and injection pain were unrelated to onabotulinumtoxinA. Regarding the systemic AEs, increased risks of muscle weakness and nausea were observed in the patients with NDOs. Other systemic safety parameters, including autonomic dysreflexia, showed no clinically relevant changes.

Because intravesical onabotulinumtoxinA injection inhibits excessive neural signals, it reduces the strength of the detrusor muscle [14,15]. Although this decreases the symptoms of OAB, it results in incomplete bladder emptying, leading to urinary retention and sometimes necessitating catheterization for urine drainage. In the patients with either NDO or iOAB, an increase in urinary retention was observed following onabotulinumtoxinA treatment, along with a high proportion of patients who had never undergone CIC previously requiring CIC.

A phase II study involving patients with iOAB investigated multiple doses of onabotulinumtoxinA injections, including 50 U, 100 U, 150 U, 200 U, and 250 U [35,38]. It was found that any dose of onabotulinumtoxinA exceeding 100 U demonstrated a higher risk of urinary retention than that with the placebo. However, no statistically significant difference in the risk was observed among the higher doses. Surpassing a certain dosage threshold increases the likelihood of urinary retention; however, increasing the dose does not further increase the risk. Our meta-analysis, which compared the commonly used doses of 100 U and 200 U across multiple studies, yielded similar results.

Regarding NDO, the patients with MS and SCI comprised two distinct groups. According to the DIGNITY study, 29.4% of patients with MS had already undergone CIC before onabotulinumtoxinA treatment, whereas the proportion of patients with SCI was as high as 84.8%, making it worthwhile to investigate the two groups separately [23,24,27,28]. After onabotulinumtoxinA treatment, the patients with MS, many of whom lacked CIC, showed a significant increase in the risk of urinary retention and de novo CIC, similar to that in patients with iOAB. However, in the patients with SCI, the majority had already undergone CIC at baseline, and no increase in the related risk of CIC was observed.

Customarily, patients with MS, similar to patients with SCI, are treated with 200 U or 300 U of onabotulinumtoxinA to improve urinary incontinence. Tullman et al. treated patients with only 100 U of onabotulinumtoxinA [29]. When observing the incidence of urinary retention alone, the patients treated with 100 U of onabotulinumtoxinA had a slightly lower incidence than that of the patients treated with 200 U or 300 U of onabotulinumtoxinA. However, when compared with patients receiving placebo, the increased RR of urinary retention with 100 U was not less than that observed with 200 U or 300 U.

UTI was the most common AE after intravesical onabotulinumtoxinA injection. The incidence of UTI correlated with whether patients with NDO or iOAB experienced urinary retention after treatment. Among the patients with NDO, those with SCI underwent CIC at baseline at an increased proportion, which differentiated their RRs of UTI from those of the patients with MS. The DIGNITY study showed significantly different incidences of UTI with onabotulinumtoxinA vs. placebo in patients with MS compared to patients with SCI (MS: 56.1% vs. 29.2%; SCI: 51.0% vs. 44.8%) [23,24,27,28]. Notably, the increased incidence of UTI was more related to the increased post-void residual volume and urine retention than to the treatment dose. Therefore, the different treatment doses did not show a difference in the incidence of UTI in this analysis.

Although urinary retention increased the risk of UTI, intravesical onabotulinumtoxinA injection might have protected patients with OAB from developing complicated UTIs. One reason for this was that onabotulinumtoxinA treatment reduced the maximum detrusor pressure, thereby decreasing the occurrence of vesicoureteral reflux, which protected the kidneys from pyelonephritis [54]. Giannantoni et al. observed that after 6 years of onabotulinumtoxinA treatment, patients showed significant improvement in vesicoureteral reflux and renal pelvic dilatation [54]. Another reason was that lower bladder pressure could enhance the bladder blood flow and tissue oxygenation, which might prevent UTIs [55]. Overall, UTIs were primarily confined to the lower urinary tract, which is consistent with the findings of other meta-analyses [56–58].

However, some RCTs did not clearly address whether patients already had UTIs or whether bacteria were cultured from their urine before onabotulinumtoxinA injection. This may distort the evaluation of the incidence of UTI after onabotulinumtoxinA injection. Additionally, different studies had varying protocols regarding whether to maintain the use of antimuscarinic agents before and after onabotulinumtoxinA injection, which could also affect the incidence of UTIs. According to our meta-analysis, the patients with NDO treated with onabotulinumtoxinA or placebo generally had a higher UTI risk than that of the patients with iOAB. Therefore, it is recommended that patients with NDOs receive prophylactic antibiotics before injection to prevent post-treatment UTIs.

Next, we discuss the potential systemic AEs associated with onabotulinumtoxinA injection. The patients with NDO generally required higher treatment doses, leading to greater concerns regarding systemic AEs. Most studies describing these systemic AEs were based on NDO. In our meta-analysis, the patients with NDO showed an increased risk of muscle weakness after intravesical onabotulinumtoxinA injection, whereas the patients with iOAB did not exhibit this phenomenon.

The effects of onabotulinumtoxinA spread from the primary injection site to the distal organs and produce related symptoms. Using onabotulinumtoxinA to treat muscle spasticity in children with cerebral palsy might carry a highest risk of muscle weakness, and symptoms could also occur in adults for other indications, such as NDO [21]. In addition to the potentially difficult patient transfer caused by muscle weakness, difficulties in swallowing or breathing can be life-threatening [21]. Nevertheless, when evaluating muscle weakness, other potential reasons for weakness should also be considered, including MS exacerbation, syringomyelia in SCI, and new-onset cerebrovascular accidents.

Nuanthaisong et al. retrospectively reviewed 13 patients with neurogenic bladder injected with cumulative doses of >360 U of onabotulinumtoxinA within a 3-month interval [59]. Four patients experienced general or extremity weakness without any life-threatening AEs, which were eventually resolved. In our meta-analysis, the doses of choice were 200 U and 300 U for the patients with NDO. The incidence of muscle weakness was low in general compared with that reported by Nuanthaisong et al. [59].

Autonomic dysreflexia may occur in patients with SCI with injuries at T6 or above. Noxious stimuli, such as instrumentation, bladder distention, or the injection itself, can induce autonomic dysreflexia. During the procedure, monitoring of the blood pressure and other vital signs is necessary for patients with high-level SCI, as "silent autonomic dysreflexia" may develop in approximately 40% of these patients [60,61]. However, in the long term, intravesical onabotulinumtoxinA injection had a positive effect on autonomic dysreflexia. Schurch et al. reported that three patients with tetraplegia and severe autonomic dysreflexia benefited from the resolution of autonomic dysreflexia with 300 U onabotulinumtoxinA injection [62].

This meta-analysis had several advantages. First, it included some recent studies published after 2015 in the analysis. This not only increased the number of patients analyzed but also ensured that the data reflected contemporary practice. Second, we systematically evaluated the literature for both NDO and iOAB. In addition to comparing the AEs between the treatment and control groups within each population, it allowed us to cross-examine the incidence of AEs between the NDO and iOAB groups. Finally, we compared whether different doses within the treatment group resulted in varying rates of AEs.

However, this study had some limitations. First, some of the included RCTs might have been terminated early owing to slow or difficult recruitment, resulting in a small sample size and high risk of bias. Second, only a few RCTs on NDO have assessed the safety profile of onabotulinumtoxinA injection. One reason for this is that the population of patients with NDO is inherently small, making it challenging to conduct related RCT studies. Additionally, the proportion of male and female patients in each study could affect the baseline status of whether patients have benign prostatic hyperplasia and further bladder outlet obstruction, which might influence the severity of the storage symptoms [63]. However, these RCTs did not separately report the incidence of AEs according to sex; thus, it was impossible to perform further subgroup analyses.

The heterogeneity in the reporting and definition of each AE is worth noting. The definition of a specific AE may vary across studies, and some studies may not provide a clear definition. For instance, in the case of UTI, the EMBARK study [41,42,44], which had the largest number of patients, and some other studies defined UTI as bacteriuria combined with more than five white blood cells per high-power field. However, some studies defined UTI based on patients' self-reported symptoms [40], whereas others did not provide a precise definition. Finally, our meta-analysis focused on short-term AEs after intravesical onabotulinumtoxinA injection. Although repeated injections are pivotal for maintaining persistent therapeutic results, the effects of repeated injections or potential long-term AEs over a period longer than 1 year are beyond the scope of this meta-analysis. In view of this, as the articles by Chen et al. and Kennelly et al. primarily discussed repeated onabotulinumtoxinA treatments, they were not included in the analysis [64,65].

4. Conclusions

The risk of UTI, urinary retention, and de novo CIC increased after intravesical onabotulinumtoxinA injection in patients with either iOAB or NDO. The risks did not vary with increasing onabotulinumtoxinA doses. Most AEs after intravesical onabotulinumtoxinA injection were localized to the urinary tract and were controlled well.

5. Materials and Methods

This systematic review and meta-analysis was conducted according to the Preferred Reporting Items for Systematic Reviews and Meta-Analyses (PRISMA) statement [66].

5.1. Search Strategy

The PubMed, Ovid MEDLINE, Ovid Embase, and Cochrane Central Register of Controlled Trials databases were searched for relevant articles from 1 January 2000 to 31 December 2022 to evaluate the safety profiles of suburothelial or intradetrusor botulinum toxin injection treatment. RCTs related to onabotulinumtoxinA treatment in patients with NDO and iOAB were reviewed. The references listed in the retrieved studies were also searched. The search keywords included botulinum, botulinum toxin, Botox, botulinum neurotoxin A, onabotulinumtoxinA, neurogenic bladder, neurogenic detrusor overactivity, overactive bladder, and idiopathic overactive bladder.

5.2. Inclusion and Exclusion Criteria

The following criteria were used to include studies in the meta-analysis: (1) patients diagnosed with NDO (including SCI and MS) or iOAB who were refractory to oral antimuscarinics or beta-3 agonists or who were intolerant to the AEs; (2) adult patients aged >18 years; (3) randomized controlled design comparing onabotulinumtoxinA with placebo or onabotulinumtoxinA at different dosages; and (4) outcomes including AEs after the intervention, such as UTI, urinary retention, and hematuria.

The exclusion criteria were as follows: (1) non-study participants, (2) single-arm studies, (3) studies not using onabotulinumtoxinA (e.g., abobotulinumtoxinA, rimabotulinumtoxinB, or incobotulinumtoxinA), (4) studies not evaluating AEs, and (5) studies focusing on repeated treatment instead of primary treatment. If multiple studies were related to the same cohort, all the studies presenting AEs were listed; however, the same patient group was analyzed only once.

5.3. Quality Assessment

To assess the methodological quality of the included RCTs, two reviewers (P.-H.Y. and C.-C.W.) employed the Cochrane Collaboration tool. The following seven domains were evaluated: blinding of participants and personnel, sequence generation, allocation concealment, blinding of outcome assessment, selective outcome reporting, incomplete outcome data, and other potential sources of bias. Each item was graded as "high risk", "low risk", or "unclear".

5.4. Data Extraction

After the two reviewers reviewed the studies, the following details were collected from each article: first author, region, year of publication, population size, sex distribution, mean age, background diseases, study design, onabotulinumtoxinA treatment dosage, and follow-up intervals. The incidence of various AEs was recorded, including localized symptoms, such as UTI, urinary retention, incidence of CIC, voiding difficulty, and hematuria. Other systemic symptoms, such as muscle weakness and autonomic dysreflexia, were also noted. This study emphasized the short-term AEs following injection. In most studies, AEs were primarily observed within 6 months of injection. If the AEs were reported at multiple time points, priority was assigned to those that occurred within the first 12 weeks of treatment.

5.5. Statistical Analysis

The statistical analyses were conducted using Review Manager v. 5.3 (Cochrane Collaboration, Oxford, UK). Because the incidence of AEs was assessed as a dichotomous parameter, the data were expressed as RRs with 95% CIs [67,68]. A significance level of $p < 0.05$ was set for statistical significance. Forest plots were used to illustrate the outcomes. The I^2 statistic provided an estimate of the percentage of heterogeneity, possibly due to chance [69], with the significance level set at $p < 0.1$. A fixed-effects model was used if the heterogeneity was not significant ($I^2 < 50\%$). In contrast, a random-effects model was used for the meta-analysis when heterogeneity was detected.

Supplementary Materials: The following supporting information can be downloaded at https://www.mdpi.com/article/10.3390/toxins16080343/s1, Figure S1: Forest plots of the incidence of urinary tract infection in patients with neurogenic detrusor overactivity due to all causes, neurogenic detrusor overactivity due to multiple sclerosis, and idiopathic overactive bladder at different doses; Figure S2: Forest plots of the incidence of urinary retention and de novo clean intermittent catheterization in patients with neurogenic detrusor overactivity at different doses; Figure S3: Forest plots of the incidence of urinary retention and de novo clean intermittent catheterization in patients with neurogenic detrusor overactivity due to multiple sclerosis at different doses; Figure S4: Forest plots of the incidence of urinary retention and de novo clean intermittent catheterization in patients with idiopathic overactive bladders at different doses; Figure S5: Forest plots of the incidence of voiding difficulty in patients with idiopathic overactive bladders at different doses; Figure S6: Forest plots of the incidence of localized adverse effects; Figure S7: Forest plots of the incidence of systemic adverse effects.

Author Contributions: Conceptualization, P.-H.Y. and C.-C.W.; methodology, P.-H.Y.; software, P.-H.Y.; validation, P.-H.Y. and C.-C.W.; formal analysis, P.-H.Y.; investigation, P.-H.Y.; resources, P.-H.Y.

and C.-C.W.; data curation, C.-C.W.; writing—original draft preparation, P.-H.Y.; writing—review and editing, C.-C.W.; visualization, P.-H.Y.; supervision, C.-C.W.; project administration, P.-H.Y. and C.-C.W. All authors have read and agreed to the published version of the manuscript.

Funding: This research received no external funding.

Institutional Review Board Statement: Not applicable.

Informed Consent Statement: Not applicable.

Data Availability Statement: The data supporting the conclusions of this article will be made available by the authors on request.

Conflicts of Interest: The authors declare no conflicts of interest.

References

1. Abrams, P.; Cardozo, L.; Fall, M.; Griffiths, D.; Rosier, P.; Ulmsten, U.; Van Kerrebroeck, P.; Victor, A.; Wein, A.; Standardisation Sub-Committee of the International Continence Society. The standardisation of terminology in lower urinary tract function: Report from the standardisation sub-committee of the International Continence Society. *Urology* **2003**, *61*, 37–49. [CrossRef] [PubMed]
2. White, N.; Iglesia, C.B. Overactive bladder. *Obstet. Gynecol. Clin. N. Am.* **2016**, *43*, 59–68. [CrossRef] [PubMed]
3. Stewart, W.F.; Van Rooyen, J.B.; Cundiff, G.W.; Abrams, P.; Herzog, A.R.; Corey, R.; Hunt, T.L.; Wein, A.J. Prevalence and burden of overactive bladder in the United States. *World J. Urol.* **2003**, *20*, 327–336. [CrossRef]
4. Lawrence, J.M.; Lukacz, E.S.; Nager, C.W.; Hsu, J.W.; Luber, K.M. Prevalence and co-occurrence of pelvic floor disorders in community-dwelling women. *Obstet. Gynecol.* **2008**, *111*, 678–685. [CrossRef] [PubMed]
5. Durden, E.; Walker, D.; Gray, S.; Fowler, R.; Juneau, P.; Gooch, K. The economic burden of overactive bladder (OAB) and its effects on the costs associated with other chronic, age-related comorbidities in the United States. *Neurourol. Urodyn.* **2018**, *37*, 1641–1649. [CrossRef] [PubMed]
6. Irwin, D.E.; Milsom, I.; Hunskaar, S.; Reilly, K.; Kopp, Z.; Herschorn, S.; Coyne, K.; Kelleher, C.; Hampel, C.; Artibani, W.; et al. Population-based survey of urinary incontinence, overactive bladder, and other lower urinary tract symptoms in five countries: Results of the EPIC study. *Eur. Urol.* **2006**, *50*, 1306–1315. [CrossRef]
7. Giarenis, I.; Cardozo, L. Management of refractory overactive bladder. *Minerva. Ginecol.* **2013**, *65*, 41–52.
8. Rai, B.P.; Cody, J.D.; Alhasso, A.; Stewart, L. Anticholinergic drugs versus non-drug active therapies for non-neurogenic overactive bladder syndrome in adults. *Cochrane Database Syst. Rev.* **2012**, *12*, CD003193. [CrossRef]
9. Majumdar, A.; Toozs-Hobson, P. Detrusor overactivity. *Curr. Obstet. Gynaecol.* **2004**, *14*, 395–404. [CrossRef]
10. Asimakopoulos, A.D.; Cerruto, M.A.; Del Popolo, G.; La Martina, M.; Artibani, W.; Carone, R.; Finazzi-Agrò, E. An overview on mixed action drugs for the treatment of overactive bladder and detrusor overactivity. *Urol. Int.* **2012**, *89*, 259–269. [CrossRef]
11. Sherif, H.; Khalil, M.; Omar, R. Management of refractory idiopathic overactive bladder: Intradetrusor injection of botulinum toxin type A versus posterior tibial nerve stimulation. *Can. J. Urol.* **2017**, *24*, 8838–8846.
12. Lo, C.W.; Wu, M.Y.; Yang, S.S.; Jaw, F.S.; Chang, S.J. Comparing the efficacy of onabotulinumtoxinA, sacral neuromodulation, and peripheral tibial nerve stimulation as third line treatment for the management of overactive bladder symptoms in adults: Systematic review and network meta-analysis. *Toxins* **2020**, *12*, 128. [CrossRef]
13. Duthie, J.B.; Vincent, M.; Herbison, G.P.; Wilson, D.I.; Wilson, D. Botulinum toxin injections for adults with overactive bladder syndrome. *Cochrane Database Syst. Rev.* **2011**, CD005493. [CrossRef]
14. Dong, M.; Yeh, F.; Tepp, W.H.; Dean, C.; Johnson, E.A.; Janz, R.; Chapman, E.R. SV2 is the protein receptor for botulinum neurotoxin A. *Science* **2006**, *312*, 592–596. [CrossRef]
15. Simpson, L.L. Kinetic studies on the interaction between botulinum toxin type A and the cholinergic neuromuscular junction. *J. Pharmacol. Exp. Ther.* **1980**, *212*, 16–21.
16. Schurch, B.; Schmid, D.M.; Stöhrer, M. Treatment of neurogenic incontinence with botulinum toxin A. *N. Engl. J. Med.* **2000**, *342*, 665. [CrossRef]
17. Schurch, B. Botulinum toxin for the management of bladder dysfunction. *Drugs* **2006**, *66*, 1301–1318. [CrossRef]
18. Gormley, E.A.; Lightner, D.J.; Faraday, M.; Vasavada, S.P.; American Urological Association; Society of Urodynamics; Female Pelvic Medicine. Diagnosis and treatment of overactive bladder (non-neurogenic) in adults: AUA/SUFU guideline amendment. *J. Urol.* **2015**, *193*, 1572–1580. [CrossRef]
19. Lucas, M.G.; Bosch, R.J.; Burkhard, F.C.; Cruz, F.; Madden, T.B.; Nambiar, A.K.; Neisius, A.; de Ridder, D.J.; Tubaro, A.; Turner, W.H.; et al. EAU guidelines on assessment and nonsurgical management of urinary incontinence. *Eur. Urol.* **2012**, *62*, 1130–1142. [CrossRef]
20. Nitti, V.; Haag-Molkenteller, C.; Kennelly, M.; Chancellor, M.; Jenkins, B.; Schurch, B. Treatment of neurogenic detrusor overactivity and overactive bladder with Botox (onabotulinumtoxinA): Development, insights, and impact. *Medicine* **2023**, *102*, e32377. [CrossRef]
21. Product Information. Available online: https://www.rxabbvie.com/pdf/botox_pi.pdf (accessed on 3 May 2024).

22. Linsenmeyer, T.A.; Linsenmeyer, M.A. Impact of annual urodynamic evaluations on guiding bladder management in individual with spinal cord injuries. *J. Spinal Cord Med.* **2013**, *36*, 420–426. [CrossRef]
23. Cruz, F.; Herschorn, S.; Aliotta, P.; Brin, M.; Thompson, C.; Lam, W.; Daniell, G.; Heesakkers, J.; Haag-Molkenteller, C. Efficacy and safety of onabotulinumtoxinA in patients with urinary incontinence due to neurogenic detrusor overactivity: A randomised double-blind, placebo-controlled trial. *Eur. Urol.* **2011**, *60*, 742–750. [CrossRef]
24. Ginsberg, D.; Gousse, A.; Keppenne, V.; Sievert, K.D.; Thompson, C.; Lam, W.; Brin, M.F.; Jenkins, B.; Haag-Molkenteller, C. Phase 3 efficacy and tolerability study of onabotulinumtoxinA for urinary incontinence from neurogenic detrusor overactivity. *J. Urol.* **2012**, *187*, 2131–2139. [CrossRef]
25. Schurch, B.; de Sèze, M.; Denys, P.; Chartier-Kastler, E.; Haab, F.; Everaert, K.; Plante, P.; Perrouin-Verbe, B.; Kumar, C.; Fraczek, S.; et al. Botulinum toxin type a is a safe and effective treatment for neurogenic urinary incontinence: Results of a single treatment, randomized, placebo controlled 6-month study. *J. Urol.* **2005**, *174*, 196–200. [CrossRef]
26. Herschorn, S.; Gajewski, J.; Ethans, K.; Corcos, J.; Carlson, K.; Bailly, G.; Bard, R.; Valiquette, L.; Baverstock, R.; Carr, L.; et al. Efficacy of botulinum toxin A injection for neurogenic detrusor overactivity and urinary incontinence: A randomized, double-blind trial. *J. Urol.* **2011**, *185*, 2229–2235. [CrossRef]
27. Ginsberg, D.; Cruz, F.; Herschorn, S.; Gousse, A.; Keppenne, V.; Aliotta, P.; Sievert, K.D.; Brin, M.F.; Jenkins, B.; Thompson, C.; et al. OnabotulinumtoxinA is effective in patients with urinary incontinence due to neurogenic detrusor overactivity [corrected] regardless of concomitant anticholinergic use or neurologic etiology. *Adv. Ther.* **2013**, *30*, 819–833. [CrossRef]
28. Rovner, E.; Dmochowski, R.; Chapple, C.; Thompson, C.; Lam, W.; Haag-Molkenteller, C. OnabotulinumtoxinA improves urodynamic outcomes in patients with neurogenic detrusor overactivity. *Neurourol. Urodyn.* **2013**, *32*, 1109–1115. [CrossRef]
29. Tullman, M.; Chartier-Kastler, E.; Kohan, A.; Keppenne, V.; Brucker, B.M.; Egerdie, B.; Mandle, M.; Nicandro, J.P.; Jenkins, B.; Denys, P. Low-dose onabotulinumtoxinA improves urinary symptoms in noncatheterizing patients with MS. *Neurology* **2018**, *9*, e657–e665. [CrossRef]
30. Honda, M.; Yokoyama, O.; Takahashi, R.; Matsuda, T.; Nakayama, T.; Mogi, T. Botulinum toxin injections for Japanese patients with urinary incontinence caused by neurogenic detrusor overactivity: Clinical evaluation of onabotulinumtoxinA in randomized, placebo-controlled, double-blind trial with an open-label extension. *Int. J. Urol.* **2021**, *28*, 906–912. [CrossRef]
31. Sahai, A.; Khan, M.S.; Dasgupta, P. Efficacy of botulinum toxin-A for treating idiopathic detrusor overactivity: Results from single center, randomized, double-blind, placebo controlled trial. *J. Urol.* **2007**, *177*, 2231–2236. [CrossRef]
32. Brubaker, L.; Richter, H.E.; Visco, A.; Mahajan, S.; Nygaard, I.; Braun, T.M.; Barber, M.D.; Menefee, S.; Schaffer, J.; Weber, A.M.; et al. Refractory idiopathic urge urinary incontinence and botulinum A injection. *J. Urol.* **2008**, *180*, 217–222. [CrossRef]
33. Cohen, B.L.; Barboglio, P.; Rodriguez, D.; Gousse, A.E. Preliminary results of a dose-finding study for botulinum toxin-A in patients with idiopathic overactive bladder: 100 versus 150 units. *Neurourol. Urodyn.* **2009**, *28*, 205–208. [CrossRef] [PubMed]
34. Flynn, M.K.; Amundsen, C.L.; Perevich, M.; Liu, F.; Webster, G.D. Outcome of a randomized, double-blind, placebo controlled trial of botulinum A toxin for refractory overactive bladder. *J. Urol.* **2009**, *181*, 2608–2615. [CrossRef]
35. Dmochowski, R.; Chapple, C.; Nitti, V.W.; Chancellor, M.; Everaert, K.; Thompson, C.; Daniell, G.; Zhou, J.; Haag-Molkenteller, C. Efficacy and safety of onabotulinumtoxinA for idiopathic overactive bladder: A double-blind, placebo controlled, randomized, dose ranging trial. *J. Urol.* **2010**, *184*, 2416–2422. [CrossRef]
36. Altaweel, W.; Mokhtar, A.; Rabah, D.M. Prospective randomized trial of 100u vs 200u botox in the treatment of idiopathic overactive bladder. *Urol. Ann.* **2011**, *3*, 66–70. [CrossRef]
37. Dowson, C.; Sahai, A.; Watkins, J.; Dasgupta, P.; Khan, M.S. The safety and efficacy of botulinum toxin-A in the management of bladder oversensitivity: A randomised double-blind placebo-controlled trial. *Int. J. Clin. Pract.* **2011**, *65*, 698–704. [CrossRef]
38. Rovner, E.; Kennelly, M.; Schulte-Baukloh, H.; Zhou, J.; Haag-Molkenteller, C.; Dasgupta, P. Urodynamic results and clinical outcomes with intradetrusor injections of onabotulinumtoxinA in a randomized, placebo-controlled dose-finding study in idiopathic overactive bladder. *Neurourol. Urodyn.* **2011**, *30*, 556–562. [CrossRef]
39. Denys, P.; Le Normand, L.; Ghout, I.; Costa, P.; Chartier-Kastler, E.; Grise, P.; Hermieu, J.F.; Amarenco, G.; Karsenty, G.; Saussine, C.; et al. Efficacy and safety of low doses of onabotulinumtoxinA for the treatment of refractory idiopathic overactive bladder: multicentre, double-blind, randomised, placebo-controlled dose-ranging study. *Eur. Urol.* **2012**, *61*, 520–529. [CrossRef]
40. Tincello, D.G.; Kenyon, S.; Abrams, K.R.; Mayne, C.; Toozs-Hobson, P.; Taylor, D.; Slack, M. Botulinum toxin a versus placebo for refractory detrusor overactivity in women: A randomised blinded placebo-controlled trial of 240 women (the RELAX study). *Eur. Urol.* **2012**, *62*, 507–514. [CrossRef]
41. Chapple, C.; Sievert, K.D.; MacDiarmid, S.; Khullar, V.; Radziszewski, P.; Nardo, C.; Thompson, C.; Zhou, J.; Haag-Molkenteller, C. OnabotulinumtoxinA 100 U significantly improves all idiopathic overactive bladder symptoms and quality of life in patients with overactive bladder and urinary incontinence: A randomised, double-blind, placebo-controlled trial. *Eur. Urol.* **2013**, *6*, 249–256. [CrossRef]
42. Nitti, V.W.; Dmochowski, R.; Herschorn, S.; Sand, P.; Thompson, C.; Nardo, C.; Yan, X.; Haag-Molkenteller, C.; EMBARK Study Group. OnabotulinumtoxinA for the treatment of patients with overactive bladder and urinary incontinence: Results of a phase 3, randomized, placebo controlled trial. *J. Urol.* **2013**, *189*, 2186–2193. [CrossRef] [PubMed]
43. Jabs, C.; Carleton, E. Efficacy of botulinum toxin a intradetrusor injections for non-neurogenic urinary urge incontinence: randomized double-blind controlled trial. *J. Obstet. Gynaecol. Can* **2013**, *35*, 53–60. [CrossRef] [PubMed]

44. Sievert, K.D.; Chapple, C.; Herschorn, S.; Joshi, M.; Zhou, J.; Nardo, C.; Nitti, V.W. OnabotulinumtoxinA 100U provides significant improvements in overactive bladder symptoms in patients with urinary incontinence regardless of the number of anticholinergic therapies used or reason for inadequate management of overactive bladder. *Int. J. Clin. Pract.* **2014**, *68*, 1246–1256. [CrossRef] [PubMed]
45. Abdelwahab, O.; Sherif, H.; Soliman, T.; Elbarky, I.; Eshazly, A. Efficacy of botulinum toxin type A 100 Units versus 200 units for treatment of refractory idiopathic overactive bladder. *Int. Braz. J. Urol.* **2015**, *41*, 1132–1140. [CrossRef] [PubMed]
46. Herschorn, S.; Kohan, A.; Aliotta, P.; McCammon, K.; Sriram, R.; Abrams, S.; Lam, W.; Everaert, K. The efficacy and safety of onabotulinumtoxinA or solifenacin compared with placebo in solifenacin naïve patients with refractory overactive bladder: Results from a multicenter, randomized, double-blind phase 3b trial. *J. Urol.* **2017**, *198*, 167–175. [CrossRef] [PubMed]
47. Yokoyama, O.; Honda, M.; Yamanishi, T.; Sekiguchi, Y.; Fujii, K.; Nakayama, T.; Mogi, T. OnabotulinumtoxinA (botulinum toxin type A) for the treatment of Japanese patients with overactive bladder and urinary incontinence: Results of single-dose treatment from a phase III, randomized, double-blind, placebo-controlled trial (interim analysis). *Int. J. Urol.* **2020**, *27*, 227–234. [CrossRef] [PubMed]
48. McCammon, K.; Gousse, A.; Kohan, A.; Glazier, D.; Gruenenfelder, J.; Bai, Z.; Patel, A.; Hale, D. Early and consistent improvements in urinary symptoms and quality of life with onabotulinumtoxinA in patients with overactive bladder and urinary incontinence: Results from a randomized, placebo-controlled, phase IV clinical trial. *Female Pelvic Med. Reconstr. Surg.* **2021**, *27*, 450–456. [CrossRef] [PubMed]
49. Engeler, D.S.; Meyer, D.; Abt, D.; Müller, S.; Schmid, H.P. Sacral neuromodulation for the treatment of neurogenic lower urinary tract dysfunction caused by multiple sclerosis: A single-centre prospective series. *BMC Urol.* **2015**, *15*, 105. [CrossRef] [PubMed]
50. D'Souza, A.O.; Smith, M.J.; Miller, L.A.; Doyle, J.; Ariely, R. Persistence, adherence, and switch rates among extended-release and immediate-release overactive bladder medications in a regional managed care plan. *J. Manag. Care Pharm.* **2008**, *14*, 291–301. [CrossRef]
51. Benner, J.S.; Nichol, M.B.; Rovner, E.S.; Jumadilova, Z.; Alvir, J.; Hussein, M.; Fanning, K.; Trocio, J.N.; Brubaker, L. Patient-reported reasons for discontinuing overactive bladder medication. *BJU Int.* **2010**, *105*, 1276–1282. [CrossRef]
52. Krhut, J.; Gärtner, M.; Petzel, M.; Sykora, R.; Nemec, D.; Tvrdik, J.; Skoupa, J. Persistence with first line anticholinergic medication in treatment-naïve overactive bladder patients. *Scand. J. Urol.* **2014**, *48*, 79–83. [CrossRef] [PubMed]
53. Reitz, A.; Stöhrer, M.; Kramer, G.; Del Popolo, G.; Chartier-Kastler, E.; Pannek, J.; Burgdörfer, H.; Göcking, K.; Madersbacher, H.; Schumacher, S.; et al. European experience of 200 cases treated with botulinum-A toxin injections into the detrusor muscle for urinary incontinence due to neurogenic detrusor overactivity. *Eur. Urol.* **2004**, *45*, 510–515. [CrossRef] [PubMed]
54. Giannantoni, A.; Mearini, E.; Del Zingaro, M.; Porena, M. Six-year follow-up of botulinum toxin A intradetrusorial injections in patients with refractory neurogenic detrusor overactivity: Clinical and urodynamic results. *Eur. Urol.* **2009**, *55*, 705–711. [CrossRef] [PubMed]
55. Azadzoi, K.M.; Pontari, M.; Vlachiotis, J.; Siroky, M.B. Canine bladder blood flow and oxygenation: Changes induced by filling, contraction and outlet obstruction. *J. Urol.* **1996**, *155*, 1459–1465. [CrossRef] [PubMed]
56. Zhou, X.; Yan, H.L.; Cui, Y.S.; Zong, H.T.; Zhang, Y. Efficacy and safety of onabotulinumtoxinA in treating neurogenic detrusor overactivity: A systematic review and meta-analysis. *Chin. Med. J.* **2015**, *128*, 963–968. [CrossRef] [PubMed]
57. Cheng, T.; Shuang, W.B.; Jia, D.D.; Zhang, M.; Tong, X.N.; Yang, W.D.; Jia, X.M.; Li, S. Efficacy and safety of onabotulinumtoxinA in patients with neurogenic detrusor overactivity: A systematic review and meta-analysis of randomized controlled trials. *PLoS ONE* **2016**, *11*, e0159307. [CrossRef] [PubMed]
58. Gu, H.Y.; Song, J.K.; Zhang, W.J.; Xie, J.; Yao, Q.S.; Zeng, W.J.; Zhang, C.; Niu, Y.M. A systematic review and meta-analysis of effectiveness and safety of therapy for overactive bladder using botulinum toxin A at different dosages. *Oncotarget* **2017**, *8*, 90338–90350. [CrossRef]
59. Nuanthaisong, U.; Abraham, N.; Goldman, H.B. Incidence of adverse events after high doses of onabotulinumtoxinA for multiple indications. *Urology* **2014**, *84*, 1044–1048. [CrossRef] [PubMed]
60. Linsenmeyer, T.A.; Campagnolo, D.I.; Chou, I.H. Silent autonomic dysreflexia during voiding in men with spinal cord injuries. *J. Urol.* **1996**, *155*, 519–522. [CrossRef]
61. Acute management of autonomic dysreflexia: Adults with spinal cord injury presenting to health-care facilities. Consortium for spinal cord. *J. Spinal Cord Med.* **1997**, *20*, 284–308. [CrossRef]
62. Schurch, B.; Stöhrer, M.; Kramer, G.; Schmid, D.M.; Gaul, G.; Hauri, D. Botulinum-A toxin for treating detrusor hyperreflexia in spinal cord injured patients: A new alternative to anticholinergic drugs? Preliminary results. *J. Urol.* **2000**, *164*, 692–697. [CrossRef]
63. Dmochowski, R.R.; Gomelsky, A. Overactive bladder in males. *Ther. Adv. Urol.* **2009**, *1*, 209–221. [CrossRef]
64. Chen, Y.C.; Kuo, H.C. The therapeutic effects of repeated detrusor injections between 200 or 300 units of onabotulinumtoxinA in chronic spinal cord injured patients. *Neurourol. Urodyn.* **2014**, *33*, 129–134. [CrossRef] [PubMed]
65. Kennelly, M.; Dmochowski, R.; Ethans, K.; Karsenty, G.; Schulte-Baukloh, H.; Jenkins, B.; Thompson, C.; Li, D.; Haag-Molkenteller, C. Long-term efficacy and safety of onabotulinumtoxinA in patients with urinary incontinence due to neurogenic detrusor overactivity: An interim analysis. *Urology* **2013**, *81*, 491–497. [CrossRef] [PubMed]
66. Moher, D.; Liberati, A.; Tetzlaff, J.; Altman, D.G.; PRISMA Group. Preferred reporting items for systematic reviews and meta-analyses: The PRISMA statement. *PLoS Med.* **2009**, *6*, e1000097. [CrossRef]

67. Higgins, J.P.T.; Green, S. Cochrane handbook for systematic reviews of interventions. Version 5.1.0. The Cochrane Collaboration. Available online: http://www.cochrane-handbook.org (accessed on 5 March 2011).
68. Deeks, J.J. Issues in the selection of a summary statistic for meta-analysis of clinical trials with binary outcomes. *Stat. Med.* **2002**, *21*, 1575–1600. [CrossRef] [PubMed]
69. Higgins, J.P.; Thompson, S.G. Quantifying heterogeneity in a meta-analysis. *Stat. Med.* **2002**, *21*, 1539–1558. [CrossRef]

toxins

MDPI

Article

Assessing the Use of BotulinumtoxinA for Hyperactive Urinary Tract Dysfunction a Decade after Approval: A Single-Blind Study to Evaluate the Reduction in Pain in OnabotulinumtoxinA Detrusor Injection Using Different Injection Needles

Heinrich Schulte-Baukloh [1,2,3,*], Catarina Weiss [4], Thorsten Schlomm [1], Sarah Weinberger [1], Hendrik Borgmann [3], Dirk Höppner [2], Kathrin Haberecht [2] and Jörg Neymeyer [1]

1 Department of Urology, Charité—University Hospital Berlin, 10117 Berlin, Germany; thorsten.schlomm@charite.de (T.S.); sarah.weinberger@charite.de (S.W.); joerg.neymeyer@charite.de (J.N.)

2 Urologic Practice Turmstrasse, 10551 Berlin, Germany; dh@urologie-turmstrasse.de (D.H.); kh@urologie-turmstrasse.de (K.H.)

3 Department of Urology, University Hospital Brandenburg, 14770 Brandenburg, Germany; hendrik.borgmann@uk-brandenburg.de

4 Urologic Practice, Kurfürstendamm 139, 10711 Berlin, Germany; cweiss@urologie-weiss.de

* Correspondence: heinrich.schulte-baukloh@charite.de

Abstract: Overactive bladder (OAB) has a significant impact on the quality of life; thus, it requires treatment that can be adhered to over a long period without undue side effects. The current treatment which uses an anticholinergic or β-3 agonist may fail to improve symptoms and has side effects, leading to high discontinuation rates. OnabotulinumtoxinA (OnabotA) detrusor injection has been approved for idiopathic OAB as a second-line treatment with good effectiveness and tolerability. This study used a visual analog scale (VAS) to assess the impact of the type of needle used for OnabotA detrusor injections under local anesthesia on the pain levels after each injection. This study included 68 female patients. We used three different needles with thicknesses ranging from 22 to 27 gauge, lengths between 4 and 5 mm, and different cuts. The sensation of pain was rated at each standardized injection location. Regardless of the needle used, the patients' perceptions of pain at the beginning of the procedure were rated as being less than the subsequent injections. Most pain sensations were rated as low to moderate. The mean pain sensation on the VAS was 2.5 ± 0.3 overall, i.e., for all patients and needles used. Statistically significant differences in pain sensation were rated only at some locations of the bladder (on the back wall and the right side of the bladder). The single needles averaged the following pain scores: 2.8 ± 0.3 for needle A (20 G, 4 mm), 2.1 ± 0.3 for needle B (27 G, 5 mm), and 2.6 ± 0.4 for needle C (20 G, 4 mm, sharp cut 15°). The 27-gauge needle caused significantly less pain, and it had no negative impact due to its length, which was 1 mm longer than the other needles. Thus, the needle thickness was a decisive factor in the patients' perceptions of pain.

Keywords: overactive bladder; botulinumtoxinA detrusor injection; needle thickness; pain; local anesthesia

Key Contribution: The thickness of the injection needle is a relevant factor in the pain perceptions of patients undergoing botulinumtoxinA detrusor injection with local anesthesia.

1. Introduction

Overactive bladder (OAB) is characterized by symptoms of urinary urgency, with or without urgency urinary incontinence, usually with frequency and/or nocturia, in the absence of a proven infection or other pathology [1]. The symptoms can be considerable and can significantly limit the quality of life for both sexes in many areas of life [2,3]. Additionally, the economic costs are enormous [4].

Accordingly, there is a wide range of approaches to treat OAB syndrome therapeutically. Conservative therapeutic measures include behavioral therapeutic approaches, such as weight reduction, caffeine reduction, smoking cessation, or fluid management, and pelvic floor therapy, such as pelvic floor training and electrical stimulation including tibial nerve stimulation [5].

Drug therapy is a primary approach to the treatment of OAB [6]. First-line pharmacological approaches to OAB consist of anticholinergic drugs, such as oxybutynin, trospium chloride, tolterodine, solifenacin, darifenacin, and fesoterodine (in chronological order). These act by competitively inhibiting the activation of muscarinic receptors of the detrusor muscle by acetylcholine [7]. Although usually effective, these drugs have many side effects (e.g., dry throat, blurred vision, constipation, and other gastrointestinal complaints), which, in addition to possible ineffectiveness, lead to a significant proportion of therapy discontinuations. They have been demonstrated to cause cognitive limitations and the development of dementia in older patients [8]. The discontinuation rate of these medications increases to 80% after one year [9].

Alternatively, mirabegron or vibegron, strong and selective β3-adrenoceptor agonists, have been available for several years and have good efficacy, a lower rate of side effects, and correspondingly better adherence to therapy [9]. OnabotulinumtoxinA detrusor injection (OnabotA-DI) has been approved for idiopathic OAB (iOAB) for a decade as a second-line treatment after unsuccessful anticholinergic or β3-mimergic therapy and is recommended in the EAU guidelines [5], becoming firmly established in patient settings. OnabotA effectively blocks the release of various neurotransmitters, such as acetylcholine, ATP, or substance P, and leads to a reduction in certain ion channels and pain receptors (TRPV1 and P2X3), which explains the reduction in contractility, urinary bladder desensitization, a reduction in urgency, and also a reduction in pain [10]. A number of studies have proven the effectiveness of OnabotA detrusor injections (DIs). Initial studies found the injection of 200 U OnabotA to be effective [11], but Dmochowski et al. conducted a first optimized dose-finding study, which led to the dosage of 100 U OnabotA that is used to this day [12].

The approval study with 100 U of OnabotA demonstrated good effectiveness in alleviating OAB symptoms and urinary incontinence, in quality of life, and in urodynamic parameters with good tolerability [13–15].

Since then, the medication has been applied to the lateral and posterior walls of the bladder at 20 different points, each with 0.5 mL of OnabotA reconstituted with NaCl (equivalent to 5 U per injection site), excluding the trigone. Most users, however, include the trigone as an injection site, and scientific data support this approach. For example, a review by Jo et al. [16] summarizes comparisons of trigone-including versus trigone-sparing injections, which indicate that including the trigone reduces the detrusor pressure and increases the volume at first desire to void. The depth of injection, intradetrusor or suburothelial, does not influence the efficacy or safety of OnabotA, as described by Jo et al. and in other studies [16,17].

For many experts, a challenge in outpatient use seems to be the fear of pain and an insufficient effect of local anesthesia [18]. Several working groups have addressed the problem of pain reduction, and protocols such as adding sodium bicarbonate to local anesthesia, reducing the number of injection sites, or exposure to EMDA (electromotive drug administration) therapy have resulted in better acceptance of the therapy [19]. The use of a rigid instrument versus a flexible instrument may also influence pain, although to our knowledge, there are no study data in this regard.

The important topic of patients' acceptance of OnabotA injections through reduced pain has been addressed not only in urology, but also in several therapeutic areas, e.g., by Nasser et. al. [20] in dermatology for the treatment of palmar and plantar hyperhidrosis. For this indication, topical anesthesia, ice, and vibration are the safest and most convenient noninvasive methods to relieve pain associated with botulinum detrusor injection. Aesthetic medicine faces similar problems: Athadeu et al. compared the effectiveness of topical anesthesia cream, vibratory stimulus, cryotherapy, pressure, and no intervention for reducing pain during and immediately after injections into the forehead [21]. There was no real "break-through" favorite in esthetics and dermatology to make the therapy more pleasant; no analgesic method to reduce pain was superior to any others. In contrast, Sezgin et al. [22], again in esthetic medicine, were able to achieve at least partial pain relief by using different needle gauges; in their study, an assessment of the multiple-injection process demonstrated a significant difference in pain level, favoring their very thin 33 G needle.

Motivated by such studies to transfer these insights to our urology field, our study aims to evaluate whether diverse levels of pain occur when using different injection needles. Therefore, our main hypothesis is that in the context of OnabotA-DI, there is a different degree of pain when using different needles available on the international urology market with different needle thicknesses, needle lengths, and needle cut shapes. The degree of pain should be determined using a VAS pain score. The needles examined in our study are listed anonymously because the user's acceptance does not depend exclusively on the pain experienced by the patient, but also on practicality and handling in use; the length, elasticity, and maneuverability of the cannula; and the cost of the needles, to name a few.

2. Results

This study included 68 female patients. The patients' characteristics in the individual randomized needle groups showed no statistical differences with regard to age, diagnosis, and frequency of injections (Table 1). Eighty-eight percent of patients suffered from iOAB. In eight patients, the injection was carried out despite a positive urine culture because the pronounced urge incontinence was the cause of the recurrent urinary tract infections. However, in these patients, there were no relevant symptoms (fever/pain) that would otherwise have been exclusion criteria.

Table 1. Age, diagnoses, and first/repeat injections of patients.

Characteristic	Overall n = 68	Needle A (22 G, 4 mm) n = 33 [3]	Needle B (27 G, 5 mm) n = 20 [3]	Needle C (22 G, 4 mm, Sharp Cut 15°) n = 15 [3]	p-Value [2]
Age					0.6
Mean (SD)	64.0 (15.9)	62.1 (15.3)	64.8 (15.3)	66.9 (18.4)	
Median	66.0	64.0	67.5	76.0	
Range	27.0–86.0	27.0–86.0	36.0–83.0	29.0–85.0	
Diagnose					0.3
iOAB [1]	60 (88.2%)	28 (84.8%)	17 (85.0%)	15 (100.0%)	
nDO in MS [1]	8 (11.8%)	5 (15.2%)	3 (15.0%)	0 (0.0%)	
Injection					0.6
First injection	40 (58.8%)	21 (63.6%)	10 (50.0%)	9 (60.0%)	
Repeat injection	28 (41.2%)	12 (36.4%)	10 (50.0%)	6 (40.0%)	

[1] Idiopathic overactive bladder; neurogenic detrusor overactivity (nDO) in patients with multiple sclerosis. [2] One-way ANOVA; Fisher's exact test; Pearson's chi-squared test. [3] Different frequencies of needles due to delivery bottlenecks during and after COVID-19 pandemic (see text).

Regardless of the needle used, there was a trend in the patients' perceptions of pain, where the pain at the beginning of the procedure (first 1–3 injections) was classified as less intense than the subsequent injections, which had a sense of an increasing sensation of pain or pain aggravation. Otherwise, the sensation of pain could generally be classified as low to moderate regardless of the needle used; the mean pain sensation on the VAS (scale of 1–10) was 2.5 ± 0.3, and the single needles averaged the following pain scores: 2.8 ± 0.3 for needle A, 2.1 ± 0.3 for needle B, and 2.6 ± 0.4 for needle C. Although there appeared to be consistent differences in pain sensation between needles (see Table 2), statistically significant differences were found only in some areas of the urinary bladder (see Tables 2 and 3). The needle that caused significantly less pain was the 27-gauge needle, whose 1 mm longer length compared to the other needles had no negative impact. Needle thickness was the decisive factor in the patients' perceptions of pain. The different pointed 15° cut of the 22-gauge needle (needle C) also contributed to pain reduction (see comparison to the 22-gauge needle (needle A) in Table 3). Needle B (27-gauge needle) showed a very mild advantage in comparison to needle C (22 gauge, pointed 15° cut).

Table 2. Pain scales (VAS 1–10) at the individual locations of the urinary bladder.

Characteristic	Overall n = 68	Needle A (22 G, 4 mm) n = 33 [2]	Needle B (27 G, 5 mm) n = 20 [2]	Needle C (22 G, 4 mm, Sharp Cut 15°) n = 15 [2]	*p*-Value [1]
LS1					0.3
Mean (SD)	1.7 (1.1)	1.9 (1.2)	1.5 (0.7)	1.6 (1.1)	
Range	1.0–5.0	1.0–5.0	1.0–3.0	1.0–5.0	
LS2					0.15
Mean (SD)	2.2 (1.5)	2.5 (1.6)	1.7 (0.8)	2.4 (1.6)	
Range	1.0–7.0	1.0–7.0	1.0–4.0	1.0–7.0	
LM1					0.15
Mean (SD)	2.6 (1.8)	2.8 (2.1)	1.9 (1.1)	2.8 (1.7)	
Range	1.0–9.0	1.0–9.0	1.0–5.0	1.0–6.0	
LM2					0.14
Mean (SD)	2.9 (1.7)	3.0 (1.9)	2.4 (1.3)	3.5 (1.6)	
Range	1.0–9.0	1.0–9.0	1.0–5.0	1.0–6.0	
LM3					0.5
Mean (SD)	2.7 (1.7)	2.9 (1.9)	2.4 (1.3)	2.5 (1.6)	
Range	1.0–10.0	1.0–10.0	1.0–4.0	1.0–7.0	
M1					0.030
Mean (SD)	2.6 (1.9)	3.3 (2.3)	2.2 (1.3)	1.9 (1.2)	
Range	1.0–10.0	1.0–10.0	1.0–5.0	1.0–5.0	
M2					0.2
Mean (SD)	2.7 (1.7)	2.9 (2.0)	2.2 (1.1)	3.0 (1.5)	
Range	1.0–8.0	1.0–8.0	1.0–5.0	1.0–6.0	
M3					0.4
Mean (SD)	2.5 (1.7)	2.5 (1.6)	2.2 (1.4)	3.0 (2.4)	
Range	1.0–8.0	1.0–6.0	1.0–6.0	1.0–8.0	
Top					0.4
Mean (SD)	2.5 (1.5)	2.7 (1.5)	2.2 (1.2)	2.6 (1.6)	
Range	1.0–7.0	1.0–6.0	1.0–5.0	1.0–7.0	

Table 2. *Cont.*

Characteristic	Overall n = 68	Needle A (22 G, 4 mm) n = 33 [2]	Needle B (27 G, 5 mm) n = 20 [2]	Needle C (22 G, 4 mm, Sharp Cut 15°) n = 15 [2]	p-Value [1]
RM1					0.6
Mean (SD)	2.6 (1.7)	2.7 (1.7)	2.3 (1.3)	2.7 (2.1)	
Range	1.0–7.0	1.0–7.0	1.0–6.0	1.0–7.0	
RM2					0.7
Mean (SD)	2.5 (1.6)	2.7 (1.6)	2.3 (1.6)	2.5 (1.7)	
Range	1.0–7.0	1.0–7.0	1.0–7.0	1.0–6.0	
RM3					0.2
Mean (SD)	2.5 (1.6)	2.8 (1.8)	1.9 (1.4)	2.5 (1.3)	
Range	1.0–8.0	1.0–8.0	1.0–6.0	1.0–6.0	
RS1					0.057
Mean (SD)	2.4 (1.7)	2.7 (1.7)	1.7 (1.1)	2.9 (2.2)	
Range	1.0–9.0	1.0–7.0	1.0–4.0	1.0–9.0	
RS2					0.3
Mean (SD)	2.4 (1.6)	2.7 (1.7)	2.0 (1.6)	2.4 (1.3)	
Range	1.0–8.0	1.0–7.0	1.0–8.0	1.0–5.0	
RBB					0.7
Mean (SD)	2.2 (1.7)	2.4 (1.8)	2.0 (1.4)	2.3 (1.8)	
Range	1.0–8.0	1.0–8.0	1.0–7.0	1.0–6.0	
LBB					0.4
Mean (SD)	2.6 (2.0)	3.0 (2.3)	2.2 (1.5)	2.4 (1.7)	
Range	1.0–10.0	1.0–10.0	1.0–7.0	1.0–6.0	
Trigone					0.12
Mean (SD)	2.8 (2.1)	3.3 (2.5)	2.1 (1.2)	3.0 (2.2)	
Range	1.0–9.0	1.0–9.0	1.0–6.0	1.0–9.0	

The injection locations and the associated pain sensations (mean, standard deviation, and range) on the VAS (1 to 10) (for the injection scheme, please see Figure 1): left side (LS) 1 + 2, left-middle (LM) 1 + 2 + 3, middle (M) 1 + 2 + 3, top right-middle (RM) 1 + 2 + 3, right side (RS) 1 + 2, right bladder base (RBB), left bladder base (LBB), trigone (TRI). [1] Based on one-way ANOVA. [2] There were different frequencies of needles due to delivery bottlenecks during and after the COVID-19 pandemic (see text).

Table 3. Pairwise comparisons of *significant* scales.

Characteristic	Needle A (22 G, 4 mm) N = 33 [1]	Needle B (27 G, 5 mm) N = 20 [1]	Needle C (22 G, 4 mm, Sharp Cut 15°) N = 15 [1]	Needle A vs. Needle B	Needle A vs. Needle C	Needle B vs. Needle C
M1				**0.045**	**0.019**	0.6
Mean (SD)	3.29 (2.33)	2.20 (1.28)	1.86 (1.23)			
RM3				**0.050**	0.6	0.3
Mean (SD)	2.80 (1.83)	1.90 (1.45)	2.50 (1.29)			
RS1				**0.040**	0.7	**0.036**
Mean (SD)	2.70 (1.68)	1.70 (1.08)	2.93 (2.16)			

The injection locations where the differences in pain sensation reached statistical significance, marked in **bold** letters (middle M1, right-middle RM3, right side RS 1); for injection scheme, please see Figure 1. [1] There were different frequencies of needles due to delivery bottlenecks during and after the COVID-19 pandemic (see text).

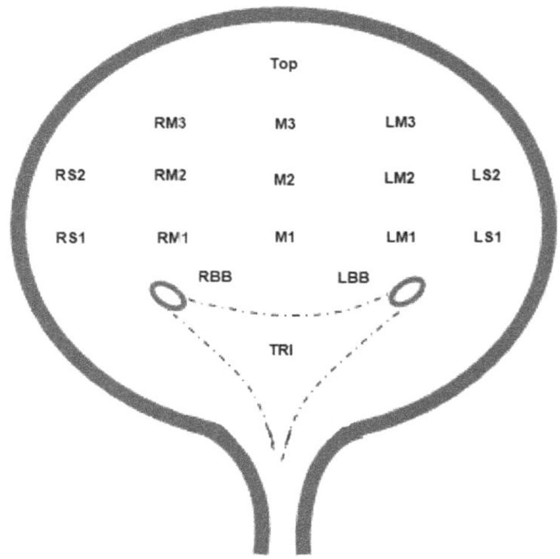

Figure 1. Injection scheme, which was reduced to 17 injections: left side (LS) 1 + 2, left-middle (LM) 1 + 2 + 3, middle (M) 1 + 2 + 3, top right-middle (RM) 1 + 2 + 3, right side (RS) 1 + 2, right bladder base (RBB), left bladder base (LBB), trigone (TRI).

3. Discussion

Many studies have shown the effectiveness of OnabotA detrusor injection for the treatment of neurogenic and non-neurogenic urinary bladder dysfunction with an acceptable pattern of side effects [23,24]. One drawback, however, is the level of pain caused by injection therapy, which varies greatly from person to person.

In our study protocol, 17 injections were carried out instead of the 20 injections recommended in the package insert, with the knowledge that a smaller number of injections might lead to an overall lower level of pain. As discussed in the following paragraph, the potential pain-relieving influence of sodium bicarbonate when added to the lidocaine solution was *not* yet considered in our protocol (although we followed this recommendation after this study). The injection pattern included the injection of the trigone. Among these injection parameters mentioned, the mean pain sensation in our study was 2.5 on the VAS of 1–10, and there were significant differences between the needles used at some injection sites. At first glance, the pain intensities in Table 2 appear (for example, between needles A and B) fairly constant in favor of needle B. However, the differences were only statistically significant at a few injection sites, which we can best explain by the underpowered study due to the supply restraints of some needles during and after the COVID-19 pandemic. However, the differences appear to be of moderate clinical importance because the inter-needle range between the average values was relatively small, namely VAS 2.1 to 2.8. In contrast, the range of individual pain perception is substantial. Pain levels between 1 and the maximum of 10 were reported, although high pain levels were reported only selectively. This is probably related to hitting a highly innervated pain point. Nevertheless, for patients who repeatedly rated the pain as being severe and stressful, the implementation of this therapy under local anesthesia should be carefully reconsidered and, if necessary, general anesthesia should be offered for the procedure.

An important question arises from our experiences and those of other users: how can we reduce the pain of OnabotA detrusor injection and thus increase the acceptance of this therapy? The literature discusses different approaches to this.

In neurology, Dressler et al. were able to show in the treatment of blepharospasm that the pain level depends significantly on the pH values of the injection fluid: by using Ringer's acetate solution instead of normal saline when reconstituting OnabotA, the sensation of pain could be significantly reduced [25].

Accordingly, similar approaches to influencing the pH of the anesthetic solution in particular have been chosen in urology, and quite different results were obtained: Pereira e Silva et al. performed a double-blind, randomized controlled trial comparing pre-injection intravesical instillations of 20 mL 2% lidocaine + 10 mL 8.4% sodium bicarbonate with 20 mL 2% lidocaine + 10 mL 0.9% saline solution. The study was carried out in women (86.2%) and men, with idiopathic detrusor overactivity (73.3%) and with neurogenic detrusor overactivity (18.1%) and, to a small extent, in patients with bladder pain syndrome. Subjects who received alkalinized lidocaine (AL) solution reported lower pain scores immediately after the procedure than those who received lidocaine solution with saline (numeric rating scale [NRS], 2.37 ± 0.31 and 4.44 ± 0.36, respectively; $p < 0.01$) [26].

Other authors were unable to demonstrate this beneficial effect of alkalinization. A randomized comparison between AL solution (10 mL 8.4% sodium bicarbonate + 20 mL 2% lidocaine solution + 22 mL sterile Aquagel) and lidocaine gel (LG) (22 mL standard 2% lidocaine gel + 30 mL 0.9% normal saline solution) showed that using AL solution for anesthesia is not superior to lidocaine gel during intra-vesical OnabotA injections [27].

Kocher et al. compared different lidocaine instillations including AL in a prospective study involving 25 patients regarding the effect on pain. There was no statistically significant change in patient-reported discomfort (using the visual analog scale [VAS]) for different lidocaine instillations ($p = 0.913$) nor for the instillation dwell time ($p = 0.14$) [28].

Another study by Steward et al. showed that oral analgesia alone with 200 mg of oral phenazopyridine taken 1–2 h before the procedure was non-inferior for procedural pain control compared to intravesical instillation with 50 mL of 2% lidocaine instilled 20 min before the procedure [29].

An interesting approach to reduce pain through intravesical OnabotA treatment was described by Ladi-Seyedian et al. in children with neurogenic urinary bladder. A comparison was made between the application of 10 U/kg body weight of AbobotA (Dysport/Ipsen) via either injection therapy at 40 sites of the detrusor muscle and leaving the drug in the same dosage in the urinary bladder for 20 min via an EMDA. The authors concluded that the EMDA group showed greater improvement with better sustained effects. AbobotA/EMDA was shown to be a feasible, reproducible, cost-effective, and pain-free method on an outpatient basis with no need for anesthesia [30]. Schurch et al. used a similar technique to improve analgesia by increasing the analgesic effect of the pretherapeutic intravesical lidocaine solution with EMDA. This procedure reduced the pain level from an average of 4 (on a 10-point rating scale) to an average of 0.5 [31].

Reducing the number of injections should reduce the pain during this procedure and lead to better acceptance of the therapy. However, Chang et al. found different results in a study attempting to reduce postprocedural pain associated with 5 versus 20 intradetrusor injections. Other than shortening the operation time, the authors found no advantages for the patients. The average pain score was not statistically significant between groups [32]. Similarly, Zdroik et al. found no significant difference in the mean pain score when comparing 10 vs. 20 injections (4 (1.5–5) for 10 injections vs. 3 (1–4) for 20 injections) [33]. Miceli et al. found that procedural discomfort related to botulinumtoxinA injection for idiopathic OAB did not differ between groups administered 5 mL/5 injections and 10 mL/10 injections [34]. This differed from the study by DiCarlo-Meacham, which found that patients' willingness to undergo OnabotA-DI again was influenced by a reduced number of injections (odds ratio = 3.8 ($p = 0.004$)) [35]. Overall, after reviewing the results in the literature, the reduction in patients' perceptions of pain through a reduced number of injections appears to be relatively small. In order to generally reduce patients' fear of the consequences of this procedure, a current meta-analysis in this journal confirms that the therapy has a low and only temporary rate of side effects [36].

To our knowledge, there are currently no studies on the influence of different needle thicknesses, lengths, and bevels on pain during botulinumtoxinA detrusor injection. Our study shows a statistically significant advantage in favor of using a thinner needle.

In summary, our study shows the following:

- The overall pain of the OnabotA-DI is mild to moderate; the VAS pain score is, on average, between 2.1 and 2.8.
- However, there are patients for whom the procedure should be performed under general anesthesia. This is shown by isolated patients who reported pain in the upper third of the VAS.
- A rising pain sensitization during the procedure appears to occur quickly, so the procedure should be kept short (via a reduction in injection sites).
- The choice of needle is of (at least moderate) importance regarding the sensation of pain.

The difference in the pain score is not a groundbreaking factor for the clinical decision regarding needle selection, as other user aspects such as length, handling, cannula thickness (which must fit through the cystoscope used), the stiffness of the cannulas, and price aspects also influence the choice of the most suitable injection needle.

However, if medical professionals have two or more injection needles of the same quality and no other advantages, they might consider to use the injection cannula with the thinnest needle according to this study.

4. Summary

The pain caused by the OnabotA-DI remains an issue that needs to be mitigated to make the procedure less stressful and increase patient acceptance. There is no clear answer, but there are a variety of nuances that may lead to a less painful procedure. The personal perception of pain among patients should not be underestimated; this is certainly important in all of the optimization efforts carried out. Factors that might make the procedure less unpleasant include the alkalinization of the anesthetic instillation, a reduction in the number of injection sites, concomitant systemic analgesia, and using the smallest possible needle gauge.

5. Material and Methods

Female patients with iOAB or spontaneously voiding patients with multiple sclerosis whose standard treatment had failed decided to undergo OnabotA-DI. They were asked to take part in this single-blind study. Each patient's written consent for the procedure was obtained. These were first or repeat injections. The study protocol was approved by the ethics committee of the Charité Universitätsmedizin Berlin (number EA4/203/22 from 9 January 2023). In accordance with current EAU guidelines, in addition to the general medical history, a sonographic residual urine determination was carried out preoperatively, a urinary tract infection was ruled out using urine sediment and culture, and a vaginal examination and a cystoscopic examination ruled out a tumor, stone, or other pathology of the pelvic floor or vagina [5].

Anticoagulant medication was stopped two days before the procedure according to the OnabotA medication information sheet. An antibiotic, generally trimethoprim 200 mg, was administered perioperatively on the evening of the injection day and the next morning. After the urinary bladder was emptied on the toilet immediately before the procedure, the procedure was carried out in the lithotomy position; after disinfection of the urethral opening, the urinary bladder was emptied with a disposable catheter (thus excluding residual urine), and anesthesia was carried out by instilling lidocaine solution 2%, 50 mL. This solution was left for 20 min.

The injection was carried out using a standardized 21 Char rigid cystoscope from Wolf with an Albaran insert and under optical control via a digital monitor, which could also be viewed by the patient if desired. The choice of needle was randomized based on availability due to supply restraints during and after the COVID-19 pandemic. Three different products were used for injection cannulas or needles, which differed in cannula length and needle length, thickness, or company-specific cut (needle A: length 4 mm, thickness 22 G; needle B: length 5 mm, thickness 27 G; needle C: length 4 mm, thickness 22 G, sharp cut 15°). The preparation used was OnabotA (Botox®, AbbVie, Irvine, CA, USA) in doses between 100 and 200 units. Regardless of the number of units, the vials were drawn up to 10 mL sodium chloride solution 0.9% in a 10 mL syringe. After 20 min of exposure to local anesthesia, the urinary bladder was filled to about 2/3 of its maximum capacity, enough to create sufficient wall resistance but not so much as to cause discomfort or pain due to excessive filling. The needles were systematically injected into the detrusor muscle at 17 locations (side walls, posterior wall, bladder roof, bladder base, and co-injection of the trigone, as shown in Figure 1). The reduction in the number of injections from 20, as described in the package leaflet, to 17, which was standardized in this study, was carried out to reduce the patients' pain burden [35]. This procedure was performed in exactly the same way in neurogenic and non-neurogenic patients.

For each injection, patients rated their pain on a VAS of 1–10 (1 = no pain; 10 = worst pain imaginable). After the procedure, the urinary bladder was emptied, and the patients were observed for half an hour post-intervention for well-being, pain, or hematuria. We did not measure the duration of effect and satisfaction with the injection in these patients as this was not the objective of this study. For statistical analyses, the mean, standard deviation, median, and range were calculated for metrically scaled variables (age, blood pressure, etc.). Absolute and relative frequencies were calculated for nominally scaled variables.

To test the three needle types for differences in the variables examined, one-way analysis of variance (with prior testing for normality), Fisher's exact test, or chi-squared tests were used depending on the variable level. For pairwise comparisons, the resulting p-value was adjusted according to Bonferroni.

Author Contributions: Conceptualization, H.S.-B. and C.W.; Methodology, H.S.-B. and T.S.; Validation, H.S.-B., D.H. and J.N.; Formal Analysis, S.W.; Investigation, H.S.-B. and C.W.; Resources, T.S.; Data Curation, H.S.-B. and H.B.; Writing—Original Draft Preparation, H.S.-B. and S.W.; Writing—Review & Editing, H.S.-B., H.B. and J.N.; Visualization, S.W.; Supervision, T.S. and J.N.; Project Administration, H.S.-B. and K.H. Each author has approved the submitted version (and version substantially edited by journal staff that involves the author's contribution to the study). Each author agrees to be personally accountable for the author's own contributions and for ensuring that questions related to the accuracy or integrity of any part of the work, even ones in which the author was not personally involved, are appropriately investigated, resolved, and documented in the literature. All authors have read and agreed to the published version of the manuscript.

Funding: This research received no external funding.

Institutional Review Board Statement: The study protocol was approved by the ethics committee of the Charité Universitätsmedizin Berlin (number EA4/203/22 from 9th available at 9 January 2023).

Informed Consent Statement: Informed consent was obtained from all subjects involved in the study.

Data Availability Statement: The raw data supporting the conclusions of this article will be made available by the authors on request.

Acknowledgments: The authors would like to thank Beate Walter from B.M. Walter Medical Writing and Katrin Wolf Medical Writing for assistance in completing the manuscript.

Conflicts of Interest: The authors declare no conflicts of interest.

References

Abrams, P.; Cardozo, L.; Wagg, A.; Wein, A. (Eds.) *Incontinence*, 6th ed.; ICI-ICS; International Continence Society: Bristol, UK, 2017.
Irwin, D.E.; Milsom, I.; Kopp, Z.; Abrams, P. Symptom Bother and Health Care—Seeking Behavior among Individuals with Overactive Bladder. *Eur. Urol.* **2008**, *53*, 1029–1039. [CrossRef] [PubMed]

3. Moussa, R.; Rada, M.P.; Durnea, C.; Falconi, G.; Betschart, C.; Haddad, J.M.; Sedgwick, P.; Doumouchtsis, S.K. Outcome reporting in randomized controlled trials (RCTs) on the pharmacological management of idiopathic overactive bladder (OAB) in women; a systematic review for the development of core outcome sets (COS). *Int. Urogynecol. J.* **2022**, *33*, 1243–1250. [CrossRef] [PubMed
4. Ganz, M.L.; Smalarz, A.M.; Krupski, T.L.; Anger, J.T.; Hu, J.C.; Wittrup-Jensen, K.U.; Pashos, C.L. Economic Costs of Overactive Bladder in the United States. *Urology* **2010**, *75*, 526–532.e18. [CrossRef] [PubMed]
5. EAU Guidelines on Management of Non-Neurogenic Female Lower Urinary Tract Symptoms. Available online: https://urowe org/guidelines/non-neurogenic-female-luts (accessed on 31 July 2024).
6. He, W.; Huang, G.; Cui, W.; Tian, Y.; Sun, Q.; Zhao, X.; Zhao, Y.; Li, D.; Liu, X. Comparative assessment of efficacy and safety o approved oral therapies for overactive bladder: A systematic review and network meta-analysis. *Int. Braz. J. Urol. Off. J. Bra Soc. Urol.* **2023**, *49*, 535–563. [CrossRef]
7. Andersson, K.E. Antimuscarinics for treatment of overactive bladder. *Lancet Neurol.* **2004**, *3*, 46–53. [CrossRef]
8. Hilmer, S.N.; Gnjidic, D. The anticholinergic burden: From research to practice. *Aust. Prescr.* **2022**, *45*, 118–120. [CrossRef] [PubMed]
9. Song, Y.S.; Lee, H.Y.; Park, J.J.; Kim, J.H. Persistence and Adherence of Anticholinergics and Beta-3 Agonist for the Treatment o Overactive Bladder: Systematic Review and Meta-Analysis, and Network Meta-Analysis. *J. Urol.* **2021**, *205*, 1595–1604. [CrossRef
10. Lawrence, G.W.; Aoki, K.R.; Dolly, J.O. Excitatory cholinergic and purinergic signaling in bladder are equally susceptible t botulinum neurotoxin a consistent with co-release of transmitters from efferent fibers. *J. Pharmacol. Exp. Ther.* **2010**, *334*, 1080–108 [CrossRef]
11. Sahai, A.; Khan, M.S.; Dasgupta, P. Efficacy of botulinum toxin-A for treating idiopathic detrusor overactivity: Results from single center, randomized, double-blind, placebo controlled trial. *J. Urol.* **2007**, *177*, 2231–2236. [CrossRef]
12. Dmochowski, R.; Chapple, C.; Nitti, V.W.; Chancellor, M.; Everaert, K.; Thompson, C.; Daniell, G.; Zhou, J.; Haag-Molkenteller, C Efficacy and safety of onabotulinumtoxinA for idiopathic overactive bladder: A double-blind, placebo controlled, randomize dose ranging trial. *J. Urol.* **2010**, *184*, 2416–2422. [CrossRef]
13. Rovner, E.; Kennelly, M.; Schulte-Baukloh, H.; Zhou, J.; Haag-Molkenteller, C.; Dasgupta, P. Urodynamic results and clinic outcomes with intradetrusor injections of onabotulinumtoxinA in a randomized, placebo-controlled dose-finding study i idiopathic overactive bladder. *Neurourol. Urodyn.* **2011**, *30*, 556–562. [CrossRef] [PubMed]
14. Nitti, V.W.; Dmochowski, R.; Herschorn, S.; Sand, P.; Thompson, C.; Nardo, C.; Yan, X.; Haag-Molkenteller, C.; EMBARK Stud Group. OnabotulinumtoxinA for the treatment of patients with overactive bladder and urinary incontinence: Results of a phas 3, randomized, placebo controlled trial. *J. Urol.* **2013**, *189*, 2186–2193. [CrossRef]
15. Chapple, C.; Sievert, K.-D.; MacDiarmid, S.; Khullar, V.; Radziszewski, P.; Nardo, C.; Thompson, C.; Zhou, J.; Haag-Molkentell C. OnabotulinumtoxinA 100 U significantly improves all idiopathic overactive bladder symptoms and quality of life in patien with overactive bladder and urinary incontinence: A randomised, double-blind, placebo-controlled trial. *Eur. Urol.* **2013**, *6* 249–256. [CrossRef] [PubMed]
16. Jo, J.K.; Kim, K.N.; Kim, D.W.; Kim, Y.T.; Kim, J.Y. The effect of onabotulinumtoxinA according to site of injection in patients wi overactive bladder: A systematic review and meta-analysis. *World J. Urol.* **2018**, *36*, 305–317. [CrossRef]
17. Kuo, H.-C. Will suburothelial injection of small dose of botulinum A toxin have similar therapeutic effects and less adverse even for refractory detrusor overactivity? *Urology* **2006**, *68*, 993–997. [CrossRef]
18. Schulte-Baukloh, H.; Höppner, D.; Hubatsch, M.; Mala, K.; Schlomm, T.; Weinberger, S. OnabotuliumtoxinA Detrusorinjektio Die "Real World" der Anwender, die "Real World" der Patienten—Update BOTUROLOGY 2022. *Aktuelle Urol.* **2022**, *54*, 55– [CrossRef]
19. Walker, N.F.; Macpherson, F.; Tasleem, A.; Rampal, T. Interventions to improve tolerability of local anesthetic intradetrus Botulinum toxin injections: A systematic review. *Neurourol. Urodyn.* **2023**, *42*, 23–32. [CrossRef] [PubMed]
20. Nasser, S.; Farshchian, M.; Kimyai-Asadi, A.; Potts, G.A. Techniques to Relieve Pain Associated with Botulinum Injections f Palmar and Plantar Hyperhidrosis. *Dermatol. Surg.* **2021**, *47*, 1566–1571. [CrossRef]
21. Athadeu, A.M.S.; Câmara-Souza, M.B.; Poluha, R.L.; Soares, V.W.H.A.; Nobre, B.B.d.S.; Manso, C.; de Almeida, A.M.; Canal G.D.l.T. Comparison of the Effectiveness of Different Methods for Pain Reduction During Injection Procedures in the Fronta Muscle. *Aesthetic Plast. Surg.* **2023**, *48*, 999–1004. [CrossRef]
22. Sezgin, B.; Ozel, B.; Bulam, H.; Guney, K.; Tuncer, S.; Cenetoglu, S. The Effect of Microneedle Thickness on Pain During Minima Invasive Facial Procedures: A Clinical Study. *Aesthetic Surg. J.* **2014**, *34*, 757–765. [CrossRef]
23. Nitti, V.W.; Ginsberg, D.; Sievert, K.D.; Sussman, D.; Radomski, S.; Sand, P.; De Ridder, D.; Jenkins, B.; Magyar, A.; Chapple, Durable Efficacy and Safety of Long-Term OnabotulinumtoxinA Treatment in Patients with Overactive Bladder Syndrome: Fir Results of a 3.5-Year Study. *J. Urol.* **2016**, *196*, 791–800. [CrossRef] [PubMed]
24. Kennelly, M.; Dmochowski, R.; Schulte-Baukloh, H.; Ethans, K.; Del Popolo, G.; Moore, C.; Jenkins, B.; Guard, S.; Zhe Y.; Karsenty, G. Efficacy and safety of onabotulinumtoxinA therapy are sustained over 4 years of treatment in patients wi neurogenic detrusor overactivity: Final results of a long-term extension study. *Neurourol. Urodyn.* **2017**, *36*, 368–375. [CrossR [PubMed]
25. Dressler, D.; Saberi, F.A.; Bigalke, H. Botulinum toxin therapy: Reduction of injection site pain by pH normalisation. *J. Neu Transm.* **2016**, *123*, 527–531. [CrossRef]

26. Pereira e Silva, R.; Ponte, C.; Lopes, F.; Pala dos Reis, J. Alkalinized lidocaine solution as a first-line local anesthesia protocol for intradetrusor injection of onabotulinum toxin A: Results from a double-blinded randomized controlled trial. *Neurourol. Urodyn.* **2020**, *39*, 2471–2479. [CrossRef] [PubMed]
27. Nambiar, A.K.; Younis, A.; Khan, Z.A.; Hildrup, I.; Emery, S.J.; Lucas, M.G. Alkalinized lidocaine versus lidocaine gel as local anesthesia prior to intra-vesical botulinumtoxin (BoNTA) injections: A prospective, single center, randomized, double-blind, parallel group trial of efficacy and morbidity. *Neurourol. Urodyn.* **2016**, *35*, 522–527. [CrossRef]
28. Kocher, N.J.; Zillioux, J.; Martin, S.; Rackley, R.; Vasavada, S.; Goldman, H.B. Patient care pathway optimization following initial intradetrusor onabotulinumtoxina injections for overactive bladder. *Neurourol. Urodyn.* **2021**, *40*, S146.
29. Stewart, L.E.; Siddique, M.; Jacobs, K.M.; Raker, C.A.; Sung, V.W. Oral phenazopyridine vs intravesical lidocaine for bladder onabotulinumtoxinA analgesia: A randomized controlled trial (OPIL). *Am. J. Obstet. Gynecol.* **2022**, *227*, 308.e1–308.e8. [CrossRef]
30. Ladi-Seyedian, S.-S.; Sharifi-Rad, L.; Kajbafzadeh, A.-M. Botulinum Toxin Type A Therapy: Intravesical Injection or Electromotive Drug Administration. *Urology* **2020**, *142*, 190–194. [CrossRef]
31. Schurch, B.; Reitz, A.; Tenti, G. Electromotive drug administration of lidocaine to anesthetize the bladder before botulinum-A toxin injections into the detrusor. *Spinal Cord* **2004**, *42*, 338–341. [CrossRef]
32. Chang, E.S.; Ringel, N.; Woodburn, K.L.; Tanner, J.P.; Bassaly, R.D.; Greene, K.; Wyman, A.; Iglesia, C. Postprocedural Pain Associated With 5 Versus 20 Intradetrusor Injections of onabotulinumtoxinA for Treatment of Overactive Bladder: A Multicenter Randomized Clinical Trial. *Urogynecology* **2022**, *28*, 518–525.
33. Zdroik, A.; El Haraki, A.; Smith, W.; Badlani, G.; Parker-Autry, C.; Matthews, C. Injection site number and outcomes of intradetrusor onabotulinumtoxinA for refractory overactive bladder syndrome: A randomized clinical trial. *Int. Urogynecol. J.* **2023**, *35*, 119–126. [CrossRef] [PubMed]
34. Miceli, L.M.; Antosh, D.D.; Nisar, T.; Stewart, J.; Rutledge, E.C.; Khavari, R. Pain Related to Intradetrusor BotulinumtoxinA: A Randomized Clinical Trial. *Urogynecology* **2024**, *30*, 337–344. [CrossRef] [PubMed]
35. DiCarlo-Meacham, A.M.; Dengler, K.L.; Welch, E.K.; Brooks, D.I.; Gruber, D.D.; Osborn, D.J.; Scarlotta, L.; Vaccaro, C.M. Reduced versus standard intradetrusor OnabotulinumtoxinA injections for treatment of overactive bladder. *Neurourol. Urodyn.* **2023**, *42*, 366–374. [CrossRef] [PubMed]
36. Yu, P.-H.; Wang, C.-C. Adverse Effects of Intravesical OnabotulinumtoxinA Injection in Patients with Idiopathic Overactive Bladder or Neurogenic Detrusor Overactivity: A Systematic Review and Meta-Analysis of Randomized Controlled Studies. *Toxins* **2024**, *16*, 343. [CrossRef]

toxins

MDPI

Article

An Alternative Approach for Treating Female Underactive Bladders with Chronic Urine Retention: A Pilot Study on Combined Transvaginal Ultrasound-Guided Botulinum Toxin A External Sphincter Injection and Transurethral Incision of the Bladder Neck

Wei-Chun Huang, Cheng-Yen Tsai * and Eric Chieh-Lung Chou *

China Medical University Hospital, Taichung City 404, Taiwan; chsh010795@gmail.com
* Correspondence: cytsai1611@gmail.com (C.-Y.T.); ericchou66@yahoo.com.tw (E.C.-L.C.)

Abstract: Background: Treating an underactive bladder (UAB) is challenging. Previously, we introduced a more precise method of transvaginal ultrasound-guided botulinum toxin A (BoNT-A) injection into the external urethral sphincter as a treatment option for patients with UABs. Although many patients experience good results, those with an UAB and excessive residual urine still require catheterization. Therefore, we developed a new method that combines transvaginal ultrasound-guided BoNT-A injection with a transurethral bladder neck incision. **Methods:** A prospective study was conducted on 16 patients who experienced symptoms of UAB and chronic urine retention. The treatment consisted of a combination of transvaginal ultrasound-guided BoNT-A injection and a transurethral incision of the bladder neck (TUI-BN). The primary objective was to assess the efficacy of this combined treatment in improving symptoms in women with UABs. **Results:** Our study demonstrated significant improvements after treatment, including increased voiding volume, decreased post-void residual (PVR) urine, and improved voiding efficiency. The frequency of clean intermittent catheterization (CIC) decreased at 1 and 3 months post-surgery, along with improvements in the AUA symptoms score and the Patient Perception of Bladder Condition (PPBC) score. **Conclusions:** Our study showed significant improvements in the surgical treatment of UABs using a combination of transvaginal ultrasound-guided BoNT-A and TUI-BN.

Keywords: underactive bladder; chronic urine retention; botulinum toxin A; transvaginal ultrasound guidance; external sphincter injection; transurethral incision of the bladder neck

Key Contribution: This study proposes a promising treatment option for patients with UABs and chronic urine retention, aiming to fulfill their dream of improving voiding and being free from CIC without increasing adverse events.

1. Introduction

An underactive bladder (UAB) is defined by the International Continence Society as a symptom complex characterized by a slow urinary stream, hesitancy, and straining to void, with or without a feeling of incomplete bladder emptying and sometimes with storage symptoms [1]. It is a lower urinary tract symptom (LUTS) occurring in up to 45% of females [1]. Clinically, a patient with a UAB primarily presents with symptoms during the voiding phase, including decreased urine flow rate, dribbling, hesitancy, and a sensation of incomplete bladder emptying. In recent years, there has been an increasing interest among physicians owing to its significant impact on patients' quality of life and the complexity of its management. Despite this, a definitive treatment that is capable of fully curing UAB and substantially improving patients' quality of life remains elusive.

An untreated UAB can lead to acute and chronic urine retention, hydronephrosis, urinary tract infections, and even renal failure, posing a substantial threat to patient well-being [2,3]. Therefore, current UAB management primarily focuses on reducing residual urine and protecting the urinary tract from further damage [4,5]. According to the 2023 European Association of Urology (EAU) guidelines, existing therapies include conservative treatment, pharmacotherapy, electrical stimulation, and surgery [6,7]. Among these treatment methods, botulinum toxin A (BoNT-A) injections into the urethral sphincter are often chosen [8–10]. However, the duration of the effect of this treatment is short, lasting only 3–9 months, necessitating repeated treatments to maintain efficacy [11,12]. Another surgical option is a transurethral incision of the bladder neck (TUI-BN); however, satisfactory outcomes have been reported in only 48.8% of cases [13]. This highlights the need for more effective treatments that can offer better relief and improve patient outcomes, especially for those with more severe symptoms. The limitations of current therapies underscore the importance of continued research and innovation in UAB treatment.

This study aimed to identify treatments for patients with UABs and chronic urine retention to achieve better outcomes while minimizing complications. Specifically, we investigated a novel approach that combined transvaginal ultrasound-guided BoNT-A and injection with TUI-BN.

2. Results

The patient characteristics are presented in Table 1. The average age of the patients was 66.1 ± 11.5 years. The mean PVR volume was 358.1 ± 192.3 mL, and the VE was approximately 24.6 ± 20.5%. Preoperatively, the VUDS was conducted, and all patients' findings revealed detrusor underactivity.

Table 1. Patient characteristics.

	Patient (n = 16)
Age (years)	66.1 ± 11.5
BMI (kg/m^2)	22.3 ± 3.1
Diabetes Mellitus	3
Recurrent urinary tract infection	0
Neurogenic disease	1
Abdominal operation history	2
Voiding volume (VV) (mL)	127.8 ± 172.0
PVR (mL)	358.1 ± 192.3
VE(%)	24.6 ± 20.5
Cystometry	
First sensation of filling (FSF) (mL)	155.8 ± 94.3
Cystometric bladder capacity (CBC) (mL)	442.5 ± 181.6
Pdet (cmH_2O)	24.8 ± 14.2
Pabd (cmH_2O)	11.6 ± 12.9
Qmax	3.3 ± 3.6
Bladder contractility index (BCI)	40.2 ± 25.1

Table 2 presents the outcomes, comparing the preoperative and postoperative profiles. The PVR urine volume, VE, and frequency of CIC all showed significant improvements at both 1 month and 3 months after surgery compared to preoperative values.

Regarding the questionnaires, both the AUA symptoms score and PPBC scores showed statistically significant improvements at both 1 and 3 months postoperatively, whereas the AUA symptoms score—QoL demonstrated a significant enhancement 3 months after surgery. Our study indicated that 88% of the patients experienced improved voiding by more than 50% at both 1 and 3 months after surgery.

Table 2. Parameters before and after the TUI-BN plus ultrasound-guided external sphincter BoNT-A injection.

	Preoperation	1 Month after Operation	*p* Value	3 Months after Operation	*p* Value
Voiding volume (VV) (mL)	127.8 ± 172.0	192.6 ± 99.0	**0.019 ***	189.3 ± 133.6	**0.009 ***
PVR urine amount (mL)	358.1 ± 192.3	118.3 ± 75.0	**<0.001 ***	76.7 ± 73.8	**<0.001 ***
VE (%)	24.6 ± 20.5	61.7 ± 17.6	**<0.001 ***	73.1 ± 23.7	**<0.001 ***
CIC (times/day)	3.4 ± 2.	1.3 ± 1.1	**0.002 ***	0.5 ± 1.1	**0.002 ***
AUA symptoms score	24.6 ± 5.3	12.3 ± 6.9	**0.001 ***	8.0 ± 5.9	**<0.001 ***
Storage symptoms	8.7 ± 2.7	7.9 ± 5.1	0.23	3.8 ± 3.1	**0.001 ***
Voiding symptoms	15.9 ± 3.9	2.8 ± 1.1	**<0.001 ***	4.2 ± 3.7	**<0.001 ***
QoL on AUA symptoms score	4.9 ± 1.1	4.9 ± 2.4	0.804	1.3 ± 0.9	**0.001 ***
PPBC	4.4 ± 1.0	2.1 ± 1.2	**0.001 ***	0.7 ± 0.9	**<0.001 ***

* means statistically significance ($p < 0.05$).

The subgroup analysis of the AUA symptoms score revealed that voiding symptoms improved at both 1 and 3 months after surgery, whereas storage symptoms improved only at 3 months postoperatively. None of the 16 patients experienced major adverse events or complications following the surgery. One patient had mild stress urinary incontinence (SUI) preoperatively, which progressed to more severe SUI during the outpatient department follow-up 3 months after surgery. Conservative treatment was attempted for 3 months, but the outcomes were unsatisfactory. We then performed retropubic sling surgery, which resulted in good voiding outcomes without obvious incontinence. There were no reports of genitourinary tract injury, major bleeding, or vesicovaginal fistulae in any patient.

3. Discussion

Currently, there is no definitive treatment for a UAB. According to the EAU guidelines, CIC is the recommended standard of care for patients who cannot effectively empty their bladders [2,6,14]. Previous reviews have highlighted conservative methods, pharmacotherapy, and surgical interventions; however, all have shown limited effectiveness in improving voiding function [2,15,16].

According to the guidelines of the EAU, surgical intervention involving BoNT-A intersphincteric injections into the external urethral sphincter can improve voiding by reducing the outlet resistance and suppressing the guarding reflex. BoNT-A inhibits neurotransmitter release at neuromuscular junctions, leading to muscle paralysis [17]. However, a drawback of this method is its relatively short duration of effectiveness, typically between 3 and 9 months, necessitating repeated injections to maintain efficacy [11,12]. Furthermore, several studies have compared the outcomes of different doses of BoNT-A injected into the external urethral sphincter. Previous research has suggested that the recommended doses for urethral sphincter injections range from 50 to 200 units, depending on the underlying condition [18,19]. Nevertheless, determining the optimal dose of BoNT-A injections into the external sphincter remains a persistent and unresolved challenge.

Reviewing previous research, a 100-unit dose of BoNT-A has been widely recommended and utilized to reduce urethral resistance and facilitate effective voiding [20–23]. Kuo et al. reported that injecting 100 units of BoNT-A into the urethral sphincter of patients with detrusor underactivity resulted in an average efficacy duration of 8.4 months, with 68% of patients achieving excellent outcomes [12]. In contrast, Jiang et al. found a lower overall success rate of 43.5% for BoNT-A 100 U injections into the external sphincter in patients with non-neurogenic voiding dysfunction [24]. Tsai et al. introduced a precise method involving the ultrasound-guided injection of 200 units of BoNT-A into the external sphincter in patients with UABs. Postoperative improvements were observed in AUA symptoms score, PPBC, and QoL on AUA symptoms score. Additionally, patients experienced significantly reduced PVR volumes and frequencies of CIC. Despite the effectiveness of this inspiring method, some patients still suffer from excessive urine retention and require CIC. This has sparked our interest in combining this surgical technique with other procedures to determine whether the surgical outcomes can significantly reduce the need for catheterization or improve CIC outcomes for patients.

Successful surgical outcomes of TUI-BN for female patients with detrusor underactivity and urinary retention have been previously documented [13,24–28]. In video urodynamic studies, Lee et al. observed that approximately 20% of women diagnosed with detrusor underactivity and urinary retention demonstrated inadequate bladder neck opening when attempting to void with abdominal straining [13]. In their study, they conducted the TUI-BN at the 5 o'clock and 7 o'clock positions. The postoperative results showed that 48.8% of the patients had satisfactory outcomes after a single TUI-BN procedure, and 60.9% of the patients were able to void spontaneously with abdominal straining, eliminating the need for catheterization. Regarding adverse events, 6.1% of patients experienced SUI, and 2.4% had vesicovaginal fistula [13].

The mechanisms underlying the efficacy of TUI-BN in the treatment of UABs remain unclear and controversial. One proposed mechanism suggests that the bladder neck is innervated by the sympathetic adrenergic nerves, which play a crucial role in the guarding reflex during the micturition cycle [29]. Previous studies have indicated that terminal nerves are densely distributed at the 4 o'clock and 8 o'clock positions in the bladder neck [30]. Additionally, urethral sphincter contraction inhibits bladder contraction [31]. Damage to the bladder neck may disrupt this reflex pathway and attenuate sympathetic overactivity, potentially reducing the detrusor muscle contractions in the spinal cord. Patients with idiopathic detrusor underactivity might experience improved voiding owing to this effect, suggesting that TUI-BN could trigger a reflex facilitating micturition [27,32,33].

Therefore, we propose treating patients with detrusor underactivity using a combination of transvaginal ultrasound-guided BoNT-A injection and TUI-BN. In the current study, the surgical approach aimed to achieve relaxation of the external urethral sphincter through BoNT-A injections and to alleviate bladder outlet pressure via TUI-BN. Our purpose in combining these two treatments was to effectively reduce the pressure at the bladder outlet, allowing female patients to void using abdominal pressure, rather than focusing on enhancing the bladder contractility. It should be noted that the effects of botulinum toxin may take 1–2 weeks to manifest after surgery; therefore, effectiveness should not be expected immediately after treatment [11]. Patients may still need to perform self-catheterization initially; therefore, it is essential for them to learn this procedure before undergoing surgery. If self-catheterization is not mastered, it is recommended to leave the catheter in place for 2–3 weeks before attempting spontaneous urination. Alternatively, the use of a suprapubic catheter is a viable option for bladder rehabilitation.

In our study, 88% of the patients achieved voiding capacity of more than 50% 1 month after surgery, and this efficacy was maintained at 3 months postoperatively. The PVR urine volume decreased significantly from 358.1 $\pm$ 192.3 to 118.3 $\pm$ 75.0 ($p \leq 0.001$ *) at 1 month and to 76.7 $\pm$ 73.8 ($p \leq 0.001$ *) at 3 months after surgery. Additionally, the average number of CIC sessions per day improved from 3.4 $\pm$ 2.4 before surgery to 1.3 $\pm$ 1.1 ($p = 0.002$ *) at 1 month and 0.5 $\pm$ 1.1 ($p = 0.002$ *) at 3 months post-surgery. Only four patients continued to require self-catheterization, while the remaining patients with detrusor underactivity were able to void spontaneously without CIC. These results are remarkable compared to previous findings. Furthermore, improvements were observed in questionnaire scores: the AUA symptoms score decreased from 24.6 $\pm$ 5.3 initially to 12.3 $\pm$ 6.9 ($p = 0.001$ *) at 1 month and to 8.0 $\pm$ 5.9 ($p \leq 0.001$ *) at 3 months post-surgery; the PPBC score decreased from 4.4 $\pm$ 1.0 to 2.1 $\pm$ 1.2 ($p = 0.001$ *) at 1 month and to 0.7 $\pm$ 0.9 ($p \leq 0.001$ *) at 3 months post-surgery. The AUA symptoms score—QoL also showed improvement 3 months after surgery, decreasing from 4.9 $\pm$ 1.1 to 1.3 $\pm$ 0.9 ($p = 0.001$ *).

We also analyzed the AUA symptoms score subgroup, focusing on storage and voiding symptoms. Storage symptoms improved from 8.7 $\pm$ 2.7 to 3.8 $\pm$ 3.1 at 3 months postoperatively, whereas voiding symptoms improved from 15.9 $\pm$ 3.9 to 2.8 $\pm$ 1.1 ($p \leq 0.001$ *) at 1 month and to 4.2 $\pm$ 3.7 ($p \leq 0.001$ *) at 3 months after surgery. These findings are consistent with our hypothesis that our approach did not primarily enhance bladder contractility in the short term but rather reduced urethral resistance and facilitated spontaneous voiding through abdominal straining.

No instances of bleeding, hematoma, or vesicovaginal fistula formation occurred after surgery. Moreover, most patients did not have any significant issues with urinary incontinence, while most of them experienced only very mild SUI, which can be greatly improved through pelvic floor muscle training, and no special medication is required for treatment. However, in our study, one of the patients had relatively obvious SUI before surgery. The patient was a 39-year-old woman who worked as a nanny and needed to commute frequently to care for infants. The patient was able to void with abdominal straining at 1 month postoperatively. Although she was very satisfied and free from urine retention, she complained of more noticeable urinary incontinence and needed 5–6 pads per day. In this particular case, after 3 months of conservative treatment with unsatisfactory results, we proceeded with retropubic sling surgery [8]. Sling surgery was performed in the mid-urethra. Under normal conditions, this does not significantly increase urethral resistance. However, when the intra-abdominal pressure increases, such as during coughing, sneezing, or lifting heavy objects, it can instantly elevate the outlet resistance, thereby alleviating the symptoms of urinary incontinence. This implies that even if patients with exacerbated SUI following our treatment for a UAB undergo any sling surgery, it will not negate the benefits of our previous treatment efforts. This is because transvaginal ultrasound-guided BoNT-A urethral injection relaxes the external sphincter, whereas TUI-BN reduces the resistance from the internal sphincter. If patients have noticeable SUI before surgery, they should be informed beforehand that urinary incontinence may worsen after surgery.

Our study has several limitations that must be acknowledged. First, the study was conducted at a single center with a small sample size, which inherently restricts the generalizability of the findings. The limited sample size may not adequately represent the broader population, potentially biasing the results. Second, the follow-up period was relatively short, which may not have provided a comprehensive overview of the long-term outcomes of the surgical interventions. Longer follow-up periods are necessary to fully understand the long-term effects and potential complications of the treatment.

Additionally, our data collection relied on face-to-face questionnaires during outpatient follow-up. This method has the potential to introduce bias, as patients may overestimate their improvements owing to the presence of healthcare providers or recall bias. Moreover, most patients in this study had complex and severe voiding dysfunctions that were resistant to conventional treatments, which could have led to a selection bias. This variability may have impacted the study outcomes, as these patients responded differently to surgical intervention than those with less severe conditions. Whether patients with mild UAB would benefit from this surgical approach remains unclear, highlighting the need for further investigations.

Finally, this was a single-arm study and did not include a placebo or control group. This design makes it challenging to determine whether the combined treatment is superior to BoNT-A 100U or TUI-BN alone. The absence of a comparative group restricts our ability to establish the relative efficacy of the combined treatment conclusively. Future studies should address this aspect by including a placebo group or comparing combined treatment with each intervention separately.

4. Conclusions

Our study demonstrated significant improvements in the surgical treatment of UABs using a combination of transvaginal ultrasound-guided BoNT-A injection and TUI-BN. This approach resulted in a notable decrease in PVR urine, improved VE, and nearly eliminated the need for CIC 3 months after the intervention. Additionally, patients showed improved AUA symptoms score, AUA symptoms score—QoL, and PPBC scores at 3 months post-surgery. No major complications were observed after surgery, highlighting the safety of this combined surgical method. These results suggest that the dual approach addresses both the mechanical and functional aspects of bladder dysfunction and provides significant benefits to patients. Although promising, these data must be strengthened by randomized blind-controlled clinical trials comparing the double treatment with each single treatment. The combination of transvaginal ultrasound-guided BoNT-A injection and TUI-BN appears to offer substantial improvements in both objective bladder function measures and patients' subjective experience. Future studies should further explore this treatment to confirm its long-term efficacy and safety in larger cohorts.

5. Material and Methods

This study was conducted as a prospective study of 16 women with UAB symptoms and chronic urine retention (Table S1). These patients underwent transvaginal ultrasound-guided BoNT-A injection combined with TUI-BN as a surgical intervention for UABs at China Medical University Hospital between January 2023 and December 2023. All patients had experienced urine retention for at least 1 year and were dissatisfied with previous conventional treatments, including alpha-blocker and bethanechol therapies. All the patients exhibited either detrusor underactivity or an acontractile detrusor. Patients with pelvic organ prolapse, severe systemic diseases (such as uncontrolled cancer, coronary artery disease, or end-stage renal disease), and an Eastern Cooperative Oncology Group Performance Status >3 were not considered candidates for surgery and excluded from the study. Additionally, patients with a documented history of previous anti-incontinence surgical interventions or spinal cord injury were excluded.

Our study received approval from the Institutional Review Board and the Ethics Committee of China Medical University Hospital, Taichung, Taiwan (DMR-94-IRB-083).

Informed consent was obtained from all the participants. All patients underwent a video urodynamic study (VUDS) in accordance with the recommendations of the International Continence Society. Age, body mass index, underlying diabetes mellitus, recurrent urinary tract infections, and surgical history were also recorded. Voiding diaries were maintained to analyze the patients' preoperative and postoperative voiding conditions. We also assessed the patients' voiding improvement using questionnaires, including the AUA symptoms score, AUA symptoms score—QoL index, and PPBC, through direct interviews conducted by the doctor before and after surgery. There were no missing values in the baseline characteristics, VUDS, or questionnaires. The primary objective of this study was to evaluate the efficacy of the combination of transvaginal ultrasound-guided BoNT-A injection and TUI-BN.

5.1. Video Urodynamics Study

A C-arm fluoroscope and a multichannel urodynamic system were used [34]. The VUDS was repeated at least twice to ensure a reproducible pressure flow trace. Data collected included the first sensation of filling, cystometric bladder capacity, maximum flow rate (Qmax), detrusor pressure at Qmax (PdetQmax), PVR—urine amount, sphincter electromyography activity, voided volume, bladder contractility index (BCI, defined as BCI = PdetQmax + 5 Qmax), and voiding efficiency (VE, defined as voided volume/bladder capacity × 100%) [35]. During the VUDS, voiding cystourethrography was performed using a C-arm fluoroscope positioned at a 45-degree angle from the buttocks to optimize the visualization of the bladder neck, urethral sphincter, and distal urethra by elongating the urethra.

5.2. A Novel Treatment: Surgical Treatment with a Combination of Transvaginal Ultrasound-Guided BoNT-A Injection and TUI-BN

Currently, according to the EAU guidelines, surgical intervention with BoNT-A urethral sphincter injections into the external urethral sphincter and TUI-BN has been approved for the treatment of UAB, although it has shown limited improvement [6,36].

Our previous study in 2023 proposed transvaginal ultrasound-guided BoNT-A injection as a more precise method for targeting the external urethral sphincter, which yielded excellent results [37]. This approach is considered more accurate, because the external urethral sphincter in women is very thin (approximately 2 mm thick) and surrounded by connective tissue [38,39]. Using ultrasound guidance, we can dynamically adjust the injection site and increase the BoNT-A dosage accuracy to the external urethral sphincter.

This study evaluated the efficacy of the described combination treatment. Additionally, these patients were monitored for postoperative adverse events using the Clavien–Dindo classification system.

The patient was placed in the lithotomy position under laryngeal mask airway anesthesia. The external genitalia were sterilized using povidone-iodine. We first performed a 70-degree cystoscopy to check for the presence of vesical stones, bladder tumors, or other lesions. An Olympus 26 F transurethral resectoscope with a needle-type electrode was used, utilizing a monopolar energy of 135 W for cutting and 80 W for coagulation. After fully distending the bladder, three incisions were made at the 4, 8, and 12 o'clock positions on the bladder neck (Figures 1 and 2). Using diathermy, incisions were made deep into the circular fibers of the bladder neck, extending distally by approximately 1.5 cm. We identified the location of the external sphincter to avoid damage. Following the TUI-BN procedure, we proceeded with the transvaginal ultrasound-guided BoNT-A injection according to the surgical steps described by Tsai et al. (Figure 3). A single 16 Fr. Foley catheter was inserted into the urethra, and 150 mL of saline solution was infused to enhance the visibility of the external sphincter. We then administered 100 units of BoNT-A into the external sphincter under ultrasound guidance, targeting the 2–4 o'clock and 8–10 o'clock positions, with 1 cc per site. Using transvaginal ultrasonography, we precisely injected diluted BoNT-A (100 units in 4 cc saline) into various parts of the external sphincter.

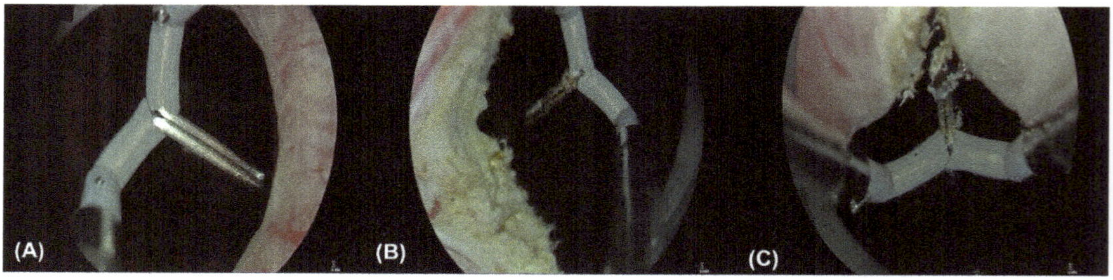

Figure 1. Transurethral incision of bladder neck (**A–C**). Incisions are made at the 4, 8, and 12 o'clock positions of the bladder neck, extending deeply into the circular fibers without perforation. The distal part of the incisions is carefully made to avoid injury to the external sphincter.

The patient retained the Foley catheter for one day post-surgery. We educated the patients on the number of CICs required based on the catheterization amount.

During outpatient follow-up, we re-evaluated the parameters using the following questionnaires: AUA symptoms score, QoL on the AUA symptoms score, and PPBC at 1 month and 3 months after surgery.

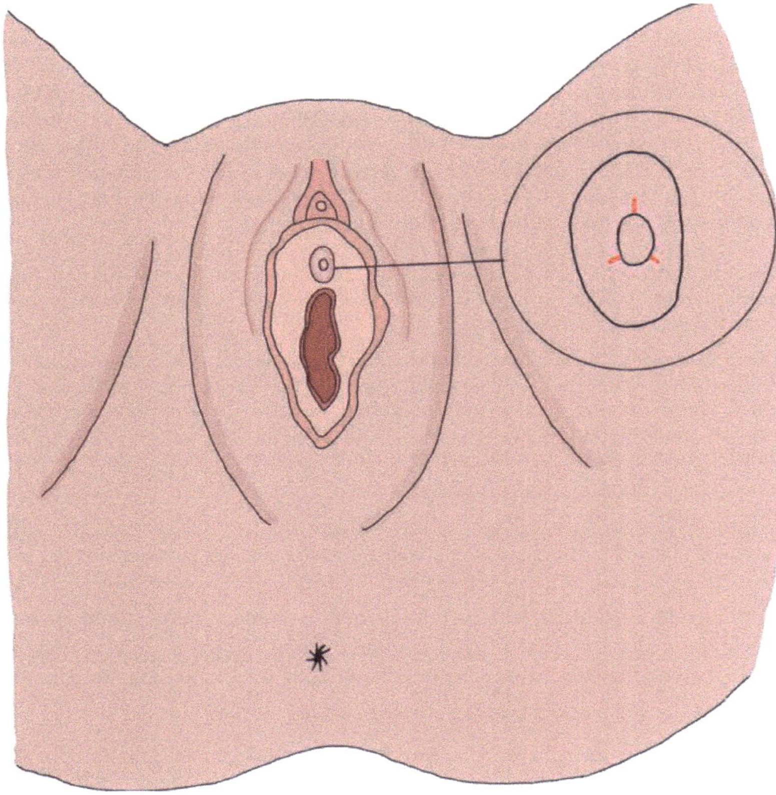

Figure 2. Schematic diagram of the TUI-BN site. We make three incisions at the 4, 8, and 12 o'clock positions on the bladder neck.

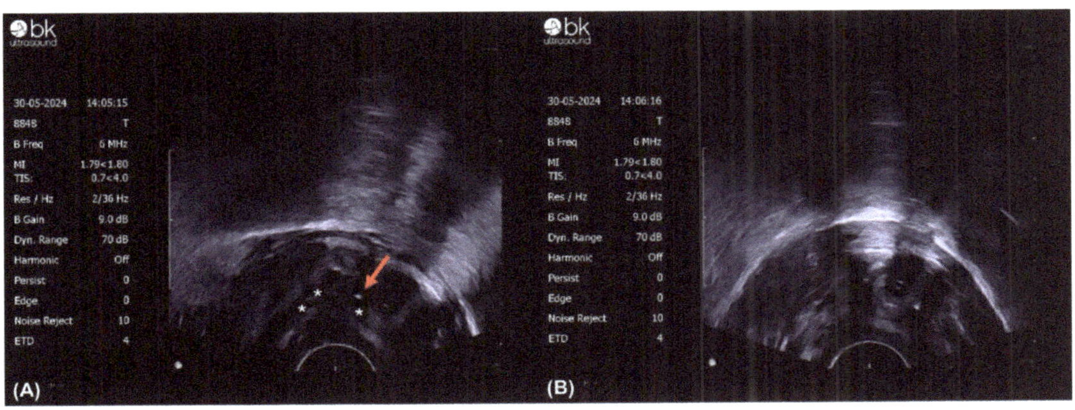

Figure 3. Transvaginal ultrasound-guided botulinum toxin A external urethral injection. (**A**,**B**). The external urethral sphincter's (dark area, marked as *) precise location can be identified through transvaginal ultrasound; injection of BoNT-A; the tip of the needle is marked by a red arrow.

5.3. Data Analysis

Demographic and VUDS parameters were recorded as either categorical or continuous variables. Additionally, questionnaire assessment scores, PVR urine volume, VE, and CIC data before and after the combination of transvaginal ultrasound-guided BoNT-A injection and TUI-BN were evaluated. Statistical analyses were performed using SPSS for Windows (version 22.0). The paired Wilcoxon rank-sum test was used to determine the statistical differences for continuous variables, whereas categorical variables were compared using Fisher's exact test. Statistical significance was set at 0.05. Postoperative complications following the surgery were documented in this study.

Supplementary Materials: The following supporting information can be downloaded at https://www.mdpi.com/article/10.3390/toxins16100441/s1; Table S1. Primary data of the 16 women with UAB symptoms and chronic urine retention.

Author Contributions: Conceptualization, E.C.-L.C.; methodology, W.-C.H.; software, W.-C.H.; validation, W.-C.H., C.-Y.T. and E.C.-L.C.; formal analysis, W.-C.H.; investigation, W.-C.H.; resources, W.-C.H.; data curation, W.-C.H.; writing—original draft preparation, W.-C.H.; writing—review and editing, W.-C.H.; visualization, W.-C.H.; supervision, C.-Y.T.; project administration, W.-C.H.; funding acquisition, E.C.-L.C. All authors have read and agreed to the published version of the manuscript.

Funding: This research received no external funding.

Institutional Review Board Statement: The study was conducted in accordance with the Declaration of Helsinki, and approved by the Institutional Review Board and the Ethics Committee of China Medical University Hospital, Taichung, Taiwan (DMR-94-IRB-083), 30 November 2016.

Informed Consent Statement: Informed consent was obtained from all subjects involved in the study.

Data Availability Statement: The data presented in this study are available on request from the corresponding authors. The data are not publicly available due to the privacy protection policy.

Conflicts of Interest: The authors declare no conflict of interest.

References

1. Singla, A.; Yamany, T.; Elia, M.; Lee, J. Female underactive bladder—Current status and management. *Indian. J. Urol.* **2019**, *35* 18–24. [CrossRef] [PubMed]
2. Bayrak, O.; Dmochowski, R.R. Underactive bladder: A review of the current treatment concepts. *Urol. Res. Pract.* **2019**, *45* 401–409. [CrossRef]
3. Wiedemann, A.; Heppner, H.J. Harnverhalt—Vom Symptom zur Struktur [Urine retention-From the symptom to the structure] *Urologie* **2023**, *62*, 1223–1233. [CrossRef]
4. Chen, Y.-J.; Lo, S.-H.; Meng, E.; Shen, J.-D.; Chou, E.C.-L.; Chen, S.-F.; Lee, M.-H.; Hsu, C.-Y.; Ong, H.-L.; Chen, J.-T.; et al. Clinical guidelines of patient-centered bladder management of neurogenic lower urinary tract dysfunction due to chronic spinal cord injury-Part 1: Pathophysiology, treatment strategy, and priority. *Urol. Sci.* **2023**, *34*, 3–9. [CrossRef]
5. Aizawa, N.; Igawa, Y. Pathophysiology of the underactive bladder. *Investig. Clin. Urol.* **2017**, *58* (Suppl. S2), S82–S89. [CrossRef]
6. Blok, B.; Pannek, J.; Castro-Diaz, D.; Del Popolo, G.; Groen, J.; Hamid, R.; Karsenty, G.; Kessler, T.M.; Pannek, J. *EAU Guidelines on Neuro-Urology*; European Association of Urology (EAU): Arnhem, The Netherlands, 2022.
7. Wang, J.; Ren, L.; Liu, X.; Liu, J.; Ling, Q. Underactive Bladder and Detrusor Underactivity: New Advances and Prospectives. *Int. J. Mol. Sci.* **2023**, *24*, 15517. [CrossRef] [PubMed]
8. Plassais, C.; Cour, F.; Vidart, A.; Bosset, P.O.; Pettenati, C.; Kennel, T.; Neuzillet, Y.; Lebret, T. Retropubic tape surgery for stress urinary incontinence: Can women be cured without voiding dysfunction? *World J. Urol.* **2023**, *41*, 2489–2494. [CrossRef]
9. Seth, J.; Rintoul-Hoad, S.; Sahai, A. Urethral Sphincter Injection of Botulinum Toxin A: A Review of Its Application and Outcome. *Low. Urin. Tract. Symptoms* **2018**, *10*, 109–115. [CrossRef] [PubMed]
10. Karsenty, G.; Baazeem, A.; Elzayat, E.; Corcos, J. Injection of botulinum toxin type A in the urethral sphincter to treat lower urinary tract dysfunction: A review of indications, techniques and results. *Can. J. Urol.* **2006**, *13*, 3027–3033. [PubMed]
11. Kuo, H.C. Effect of botulinum a toxin in the treatment of voiding dysfunction due to detrusor underactivity. *Urology* **2003**, *61*, 55 [CrossRef]
12. Kuo, H.C. Comparison of the therapeutic effects of urethralinjections of 50 and 100 units of botulinum A toxin forvoiding dysfunction. *Tzu Chi Med. J.* **2007**, *19*, 134–138. [CrossRef]

3. Lee, Y.K.; Kuo, H.C. Therapeutic Efficacy and Quality of Life Improvement in Women with Detrusor Underactivity Following Transurethral Incision of the Bladder Ne. *Urol. Sci.* **2019**, *30*, 266. [CrossRef]
4. Arlandis, S.; Bø, K.; Cobussen-Boekhorst, H.; Costantini, E.; de Heide, M.; Farag, F.; Groen, J.; Karavitakis, M.; Lapitan, M.C.; Manso, M.; et al. European Association of Urology Guidelines on the Management of Female Non-neurogenic Lower Urinary Tract Symptoms. Part 2: Underactive Bladder, Bladder Outlet Obstruction, and Nocturia. *Eur. Urol.* **2022**, *82*, 60–70. [CrossRef]
5. Chang, Y.H.; Siu, J.J.; Hsiao, P.J.; Chang, C.H.; Chou, E.C. Review of underactive bladder. *J. Formos. Med. Assoc.* **2018**, *117*, 178–184. [CrossRef] [PubMed]
6. Gani, J.; Hennessey, D. The underactive bladder: Diagnosis and surgical treatment options. *Transl. Androl. Urol.* **2017**, *6*, S186–S195. [CrossRef]
7. Chancellor, M.B.; Fowler, C.J.; Apostolidis, A.; de Groat, W.C.; Smith, C.P.; Somogyi, G.T.; Aoki, K.R. Drug Insight: Biological effects of botulinum toxin A in the lower urinary tract. *Nat. Clin. Pract. Urol.* **2008**, *5*, 319–328. [CrossRef]
8. Kao, Y.L.; Huang, K.H.; Kuo, H.C.; Ou, Y.C. The Therapeutic Effects and Pathophysiology of Botulinum Toxin A on Voiding Dysfunction Due to Urethral Sphincter Dysfunction. *Toxins* **2019**, *11*, 728. [CrossRef]
9. Kao, Y.L.; Chen, J.T.; Chen, S.L.; Shao, I.H.; Wang, C.C.; Chiang, I.N.; Hsu, Y.C.; Lee, K.H.; Lee, W.C.; Yeh, T.C.; et al. Clinical guidelines of patient-centered bladder management of neurogenic lower urinary tract dysfunction due to chronic spinal cord injury—Part 2: Conservative and minimally invasive treatment. *Urol. Sci.* **2023**, *34*, 10–17. [CrossRef]
0. Schurch, B.; Hauri, D.; Rodic, B.; Curt, A.; Meyer, M.; Rossier, A.B. Botulinum-A toxin as a treatment ofdetrusor-sphincter dyssynergia: A prospective study in 24 spinal cord injurypatients. *J. Urol.* **1996**, *155*, 1023–1029. [CrossRef]
1. Kuo, H.C. Botulinum A toxin urethral injection for the treatment of lowerurinary tract dysfunction. *J. Urol.* **2003**, *170*, 1908–1912. [CrossRef]
2. Phelan, M.W.; Franks, M.; Somogyi, G.T.; Yokoyama, T.; Fraser, M.O.; Lavelle, J.P.; Yoshimura, N.; Chancellor, M.B. Botulinum toxin urethral sphincterinjection to restore bladder emptying in men and women with voidingdysfunction. *J. Urol.* **2001**, *165*, 1107–1110. [CrossRef]
3. Petit, H.; Gallien, P.; de Sèze, M.-P.; Joseph, P.-A.; Mazaux, J.-M.; Barat, M. Botulinum A Toxin and Detrusor Sphincter Dyssynergia: A Double-Blind Lidocaine-Controlled Study in 13 Patients with Spinal Cord Disease. *Eur. Urol.* **2002**, *42*, 56–62.
4. Jiang, Y.H.; Wang, C.C.; Kuo, H.C. OnabotulinumtoxinA Urethral Sphincter Injection as Treatment for Non-neurogenic Voiding Dysfunction—A Randomized, Double-Blind, Placebo-Controlled Study. *Sci. Rep.* **2016**, *6*, 38905. [CrossRef]
5. Jhang, J.F.; Jiang, Y.H.; Lee, C.L.; Kuo, H.C. Long-term follow up and predictive factors for successful outcome of transurethral incision of the bladder neck in women with detrusor underactivity. *J. Formos. Med. Assoc.* **2016**, *115*, 807–813. [CrossRef]
6. Kuo, H.C. Recovery of detrusor function after urethral botulinum A toxin injection in patients with idiopathic low detrusor contractility and voiding dysfunction. *Urology* **2007**, *69*, 57–61. [CrossRef]
7. Jhang, J.F.; Jiang, Y.H.; Kuo, H.C. Transurethral incision of the bladder neck improves voiding efficiency in female patients with detrusor underactivity. *Int. Urogynecol. J.* **2014**, *25*, 671–676. [CrossRef] [PubMed]
8. Kuo, H.C. Videourodynamic Precision Diagnosis and Treatment of Lower Urinary Tract Symptoms in Women. *Urol. Sci.* **2021**, *32*, 94–101. [CrossRef]
9. Junginger, B.; Baessler, K.; Sapsford, R.; Hodges, P.W. Effect of abdominal and pelvic floor tasks on muscle activity, abdominal pressure and bladder neck. *Int. Urogynecol. J.* **2010**, *21*, 69–77. [CrossRef] [PubMed]
0. Ball, T.P., Jr.; Teichman, J.M.; Sharkey, F.E.; Rogenes, V.J.; Adrian, E.K. Terminal nerve distribution to the urethra and bladder neck: Considerations in the management of stress urinary incontinence. *J. Urol.* **1997**, *158*, 827–829. [CrossRef]
1. Thor, K.B.; de Groat, W.C. Neural control of the female urethral and anal rhabdosphincters and pelvic floor muscles. *Am. J. Physiol. Regul. Integr. Comp. Physiol.* **2010**, *299*, R416–R438. [CrossRef]
2. Jiang, Y.H.; Lee, C.L.; Jhang, J.F.; Kuo, H.C. Current pharmacological and surgical treatment of underactive bladder. *Ci Ji Yi Xue Za Zhi* **2017**, *29*, 187–191. [PubMed]
3. Ke, Q.S.; Kuo, H.C. Transurethral incision of the bladder neck to treat bladder neck dysfunction and voiding dysfunction in patients with high-level spinal cord injuries. *Neurourol. Urodyn.* **2010**, *29*, 748–752. [CrossRef]
4. Gammie, A.; Clarkson, B.; Constantinou, C.; Damaser, M.; Drinnan, M.; Geleijnse, G.; Griffiths, D.; Rosier, P.; Schäfer, W.; Van Mastrigt, R. International continence society guidelines on urodynamic equipment performance. *Neurourol. Urodynamics* **2014**, *33*, 370–379. [CrossRef]
5. Abrams, P. Bladder outlet obstruction index, bladder contractility index and bladder voiding efficiency: Three simple indices to define bladder voiding function. *BJU Int.* **1999**, *84*, 14–15. [CrossRef] [PubMed]
6. Chen, S.F.; Jhang, J.F.; Jiang, Y.H.; Kuo, H.C. Treatment outcomes of detrusor underactivity in women based on clinical and videourodynamic characteristics. *Int. Urol. Nephrol.* **2022**, *54*, 1215–1223. [CrossRef] [PubMed]
7. Tsai, C.Y.; Yeh, Y.H.; Tsai, L.H.; Chou, E.C. The Efficacy of Transvaginal Ultrasound-Guided BoNT-A External Sphincter Injection in Female Patients with Underactive Bladder. *Toxins* **2023**, *15*, 199. [CrossRef] [PubMed]

38. Macura, K.J.; Genadry, R.; Borman, T.L.; Mostwin, J.L.; Lardo, A.C.; Bluemke, D.A. Evaluation of the female urethra wit intraurethral magnetic resonance imaging. *J. Magn. Reason. Imaging* **2004**, *20*, 153–159. [CrossRef]
39. Chaudhari, V.V.; Patel, M.K.; Douek, M.; Raman, S.S. MR imaging and US of female urethral and periurethral disease. *Radiographic* **2010**, *30*, 1857–1874. [CrossRef]

toxins

MDPI

Article

Assessing the Use of BotulinumtoxinA for Hyperactive Urinary Tract Dysfunction a Decade After Approval: General Versus Local Anesthesia for BotulinumtoxinA Detrusor Injection

Heinrich Schulte-Baukloh [1,2,3,*], Apostolos Apostolidis [4], Catarina Weiss [5], Thorsten Schlomm [1], Sarah Weinberger [1], Dirk Höppner [2], Kathrin Haberecht [2], Carsten Waskow [2], Hendrik Borgmann [3], Jörg Neymeyer [1] and Bernhard Ralla [1]

1 Department of Urology, Charité—University Hospital Berlin, 12203 Berlin, Germany
2 Urologic Practice Turmstrasse, Mitte/Moabit, 10551 Berlin, Germany
3 Department of Urology, University Hospital Brandenburg, 14770 Brandenburg, Germany
4 2nd Department of Urology, Aristotle University of Thessaloniki, 56403 Thessaloniki, Greece
5 Urologic Practice Kurfürstendamm, Charlottenburg, 10711 Berlin, Germany
* Correspondence: heinrich.schulte-baukloh@charite.de; Tel.: +49-(0)176-490-55-620

Abstract: Background: The onabotulinumtoxinA detrusor injection (OnabotA DI) was approved a decade ago for the treatment of patients with idiopathic overactive bladder (iOAB) or neurogenic detrusor overactivity (nDO) dysfunction who had not been treated successfully otherwise. The procedure is usually performed under local anesthesia (LA), and various approaches have been investigated to make the procedure as painless as possible. We examined the level of anxiety and pain experienced by patients who wanted to have the procedure performed under LA or general anesthesia (GA). **Material and Methods**: Patients scheduled for OnabotA DI were able to choose the anesthesia procedure (LA or GA). The Amsterdam Preoperative Anxiety and Information Scale (APAIS) was used to grade anxiety before anesthesia or before the procedure itself. Intra- and postoperative pain was determined using the Visual Analogue Scale (VAS). Various established questionnaires (including the Urinary Distress Inventory UDI-6), as well as a postoperative satisfaction questionnaire, were used to evaluate the success of the therapy. **Results**: In total, 104 patients (93 F, 11 M; age 64.0 (22–89) years; 80× iOAB, 24× nDO) were evaluated. OnabotA-DI was performed with LA in 72 patients and GA in 32. Stratified by first versus repeat injection in the LA group, there was a significant decrease in the Anxiety Score in the first vs. repeat injection group ($p = 0.038$). The LA group showed higher concerns in the anesthesia questions of the Amsterdam Preoperative Anxiety and Information Scale (APAIS) than the GA group (OR: 0.29, 95%CI: 0.02–1.74). The VAS Pain Score during the procedure was significantly lower in the GA group compared to the LA group (LA: 3.3 ± 2.2, GA group 1.5 ± 1.5; $p < 0.001$). There were no differences in the success of therapy. Despite the fear and pain, patients preferred LA to GA. **Conclusions**: This study shows that the anxiety and pain burden of patients undergoing OnabotA-DI under LA is significant in comparison to GA during the first injection, but insignificant for following injections. Overall, LA is favored over GA.

Keywords: overactive bladder; neurogenic bladder; botulinumtoxinA detrusor injection; pain; anxiety; local anesthesia; general anesthesia

Key Contribution: Despite higher levels of fear and pain, the botulinumtoxinA detrusor injection carried out under local anesthesia is preferred over the procedure under general anesthesia.

1. Introduction

OnabotulinumtoxinA detrusor injection (OnabotA-DI) is used for various disorders associated with an hyperactive lower urinary tract, such as idiopathic overactive bladder (iOAB) and neurogenic detrusor overactivity (nDO) in multiple sclerosis or spinal cord patients, as well as nDO of other origins, such as post-stroke or Parkinson's disease [1], and children with spina bifida [2], or lower urinary tract symptoms due to benign prostatic hyperplasia [3], interstitial cystitis [4], and dysfunctional voiding [5]. The Food and Drug Administration (FDA) approved OnabotA-DI for nDO in multiple sclerosis (MS) patients or subcervical spinal cord patients adults or children >5 years of age and as a second-line treatment of iOAB with symptoms of urge urinary incontinence, urgency, and frequency in adults who have an inadequate response to or are intolerant of an anticholinergic medication [6].

Briefly, Botulinum-neurotoxinA (BoNT/A) cleaves SNAP-25 (synaptosomal-associated protein with a molecular weight of 25 kDa), which is, together with synaptobrevin (a vesicle-associated membrane protein) and syntaxin, an essential component of the SNARE (soluble N-ethylmaleimide-sensitive fusion attachment protein receptor) complex of the neuronal end plate. This leads to blockage of the fusion of the transmitter-containing vesicles with the presynaptic membrane. By inhibiting the release of various transmitters (e.g., acetylcholine, adenosine-triphosphate (ATP), calcitonin gene-related peptide (CGRP), or glutamate), this has an inhibitory effect on the signal transduction of efferent and afferent neuronal pathways. When injected in the bladder, both the motor cholinergic—via detrusor muscarinic receptors—and the sensory purinergic (via P2X3 receptors) signaling pathways are hindered, further to a decrease in the suburothelial afferent receptor transient receptor potential vanilloid 1 (TRPV1). An indirect way of reducing the latter receptors through inhibition of the bladder nerve growth factor is suspected. This afferent desensitization effect explains the good impact not only in patients with detrusor overactivity but also in patients with increased bladder sensation or bladder pain in interstitial cystitis/bladder pain syndrome [7]. Retrograde transfer of the toxin to the central nervous system after bladder injection also seems plausible, and thus a central effect on bladder control has been proposed as an additional mechanism of action [8].

After an initial dose-finding study [9], relief of hyperactive bladder dysfunction by OnabotA-DI for iOAB and nDO was shown in several studies [10–15]. In the approval studies [10], as well as in follow-up studies [11], regarding OnabotA-DI for iOAB, there was a reduction in daily incontinence episodes in the OnabotA group compared to the placebo group, a corresponding reduction in the mean number of daily micturition, urgency, and nocturia episodes, and a significant, positive influence on the patients' quality of life [15]. Recent data (GRACE-study [16]) also confirm these results in the real world, as well as impacting the use of incontinence aids and medication [17]; there was also a significantly lower incidence of urinary retention requiring catheterization, in contrast to 5.8% in the approval study [10]. Patients with nDO showed a significant reduction in urinary incontinence, an increase in bladder capacity, an increase in urodynamic reflex volume, and a reduction in detrusor overactivity after 200 or 300 U of OnabotA DI [13]. Side effects in both nDO and iOAB were summarized in a recent meta-analysis [18].

The procedure of OnabotA-DI is carried out cystoscopically, usually under local anesthesia (LA), by injecting OnabotA dissolved in sodium chloride into approximately 20 locations of the detrusor muscle, including the side walls, the posterior wall, and the base of the bladder. Most surgeons include the trigonum, contrary to the manufacturer's instructions. A needle with a length of 4–5 mm and a diameter usually of 22–27 gauge is used for the injection.

However, for many patients, a major hurdle to choosing this therapy to relieve their symptoms is fear of the invasive procedure, cystoscopy, multiple injections, and side effects such as urinary retention. In particular, pain is an obstacle for patients who may undergo this therapy for the first or repeated times, and surgeons alike might have concerns about inadequate local anesthesia [19]. Accordingly, there are a number of approaches to positively influence the pain of injection therapy. For example, fewer injections are carried out than the 20 injections specified by the manufacturer, apparently without any loss of effectiveness [20] (but there are also contradictory results in terms of pain diminution by reducing the injection number [21]). Sodium bicarbonate may be added to the anesthesiological lidocaine solution because increasing the pH value increases the permeability of the urinary bladder mucosa for the LA, thus contributing to a reduction in pain [22]. In rare cases, electromotive drug administration has also been used successfully [23].

Due to the fear of pain during the procedure, there are patients who prefer the procedure to be carried out under general anesthesia (GA). In order to obtain a clearer picture of the stress on patients under LA versus GA, we examined whether patients generally prefer to undergo OnabotA DI under LA or GA, what the different levels of anxiety are before anesthesia or before the surgical procedure, what the different levels of pain are, whether there are differences in the treatment outcome, and which form of anesthesia is preferred by patients who experienced both forms of anesthesia.

2. Results

In total, 104 patients (93 F, 11 M; mean age: 64.0 (22–89) years, median 68 years) were evaluated (Figure 1); 80 patients had iOAB and 24 had nDO. OnabotA DI was performed in 72 patients with LA and in 32 with GA. The groups were comparable with regard to age and type of bladder dysfunction. Male patients decided significantly more often to have the procedure performed under GA (Table 1).

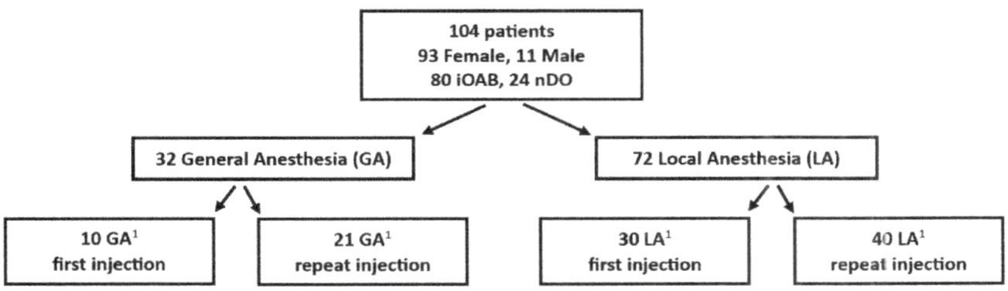

Figure 1. Overview of the study protocol ([1] difference to 104: n = 3 unknown whether first or repeated injection).

Table 1. Basic demographics, diagnosis, and dosage of OnabotulinumtoxinA (OnabotA); GA = general anesthesia, LA = local anesthesia; standard deviation (SD); male (M), female (F); idiopathic overactive bladder (iOAB), neurogenic detrusor overactivity (nDO); [1] n; [2] Wilcoxon rank-sum test; Fisher's exact test; Pearson's Chi-squared test.

Characteristic	Overall, n = 104 [1]	GA, n = 32 [1]	LA, n = 72 [1]	p-Value [2]
Age				0.2
Mean (SD)	64.0 (13.9)	61.9 (12.6)	65.0 (14.4)	
Median	67.5	62.0	68.0	
Range	22.0–89.0	32.0–80.0	22.0–89.0	
Gender				**<0.001**
M	11 (10.6%)	10 (31.2%)	1 (1.4%)	
F	93 (89.4%)	22 (68.8%)	71 (98.6%)	
Diagnosis				0.8
OAB	80 (76.9%)	24 (75.0%)	56 (77.8%)	
nDO	24 (23.1%)	8 (25.0%)	16 (22.2%)	
Dosage				0.9
100	79 (76.7%)	25 (78.1%)	54 (76.1%)	
150	9 (8.7%)	2 (6.2%)	7 (9.9%)	
200	15 (14.6%)	5 (15.6%)	10 (14.1%)	

The following results were found regarding undergoing OnabotA DI under LA versus GA. The preoperative APAIS showed no significant differences in the sum score between the two groups in the category of anxiety in the overall cohort (initial and repeat injections together; total score LA group 6.5 ± 3.5 vs. GA group 6.0 ± 3.6; p = 0.4). However, individual questions in the APAIS questionnaire showed that the question about fear of anesthesia in the LA group was given a score ≥ 4 (very great or extreme fear) by one in ten patients (10.3%), in contrast to 3.2% in the GA group (odds ratio (OR): 0.29, 95% CI: 0.02–1.74). The situation was similar (score ≥ 4) for "being concerned about the anesthesia" (LA vs. GA: 7.8% vs. 3.2%; OR: 0.39, 95% CI: 0.02–2.58). The "Desire for Information Score", a query in the APAIS questionnaire that assesses the need for the extent of explanation/information, was not significantly different (Table 2). Similarly, fear of the OnabotA-DI procedure itself was not different between groups.

Table 2. Anxiety Score and Desire for Information Score of the APAIS Questionnaire (Amsterdam Preoperative Anxiety and Information Scale).

Characteristic	Overall, n = 104	GA, n = 32	LA, n = 72	p-Value
Anxiety Score				0.4
Mean (SD)	6.3 (3.6)	6.0 (3.6)	6.5 (3.5)	
Median	5.0	4.0	5.0	
Range	4.0–16.0	4.0–16.0	4.0–16.0	
Missing	18	3	15	
Desire for Information Score				0.5
Mean (SD)	4.2 (2.4)	4.5 (2.6)	4.1 (2.4)	
Median	4.0	4.0	4.0	
Range	0.0–9.0	0.0–9.0	0.0–8.0	
Missing	1	1	0	

However, when stratified according to whether the procedure was performed for the first time (LA group: 30; GA group: 10) or the repeated time (LA group: 40; GA group: 21; unknown: 3), the Anxiety Score in the LA group at the first injection was significantly higher than in the GA group (8.7 ± 4.2 vs. 5.9 ± 3.0; p = 0.038; Table 3, visualized in Figure 2). In the LA group, the Anxiety Score for the repeat injection was highly significantly lower than at the first injection (8.7 ± 4.2 vs. 4.8 ± 1.7; p < 0.001). The Anxiety Score for the repeat injection did not differ significantly between the LA and GA groups (p = 0.2; Table 3).

Table 3. Anxiety Score and Desire for Information Score of the APAIS Questionnaire (Amsterdam Preoperative Anxiety and Information Scale) stratified for first versus repeat injection. Significant differences are shown in **bold** numbers.

	First Injection			Repeated Injection		
Characteristic	GA, n = 10	LA, n = 30	p-Value	GA, n = 21	LA, n = 40	p-Value
Anxiety Score			0.038 [1]			0.2
Mean (SD)	**5.9 (3.0)**	**8.7 (4.2)** [2]		6.2 (4.0)	4.8 (1.7) [2]	
Median	4.0	8.0		4.0	4.0	
Range	4.0–13.0	4.0–16.0		4.0–16.0	4.0–12.0	
Desire for Information Score			0.6			0.7 [1]
Mean (SD)	5.0 (2.6)	4.4 (2.6)		4.3 (2.7)	3.9 (2.1)	
Median	5.0	4.0		4.0	4.0	
Range	2.0–8.0	0.0–8.0		0.0–9.0	0.0–8.0	

[1] Wilcoxon rank sum test. [2] Difference in LA group Anxiety Score first vs. repeat injection: p < 0.001.

In the GA group, fear scores were not significantly different between the first and repeated injections (5.9 ± 3.0 vs. 6.2 ± 4.0, p = 0.816). However, there was a significant difference in the Pain Score during the procedure (Figure 3). Patients in the GA group tended to report that the procedure was more unpleasant within the first 24 h after the procedure than those in the LA group (GA group: 2.9 ± 2.4 vs. LA group: 2.2 ± 1.7, n.s.). Information about the most severe postoperative pain or the use of painkillers was not significantly different between groups.

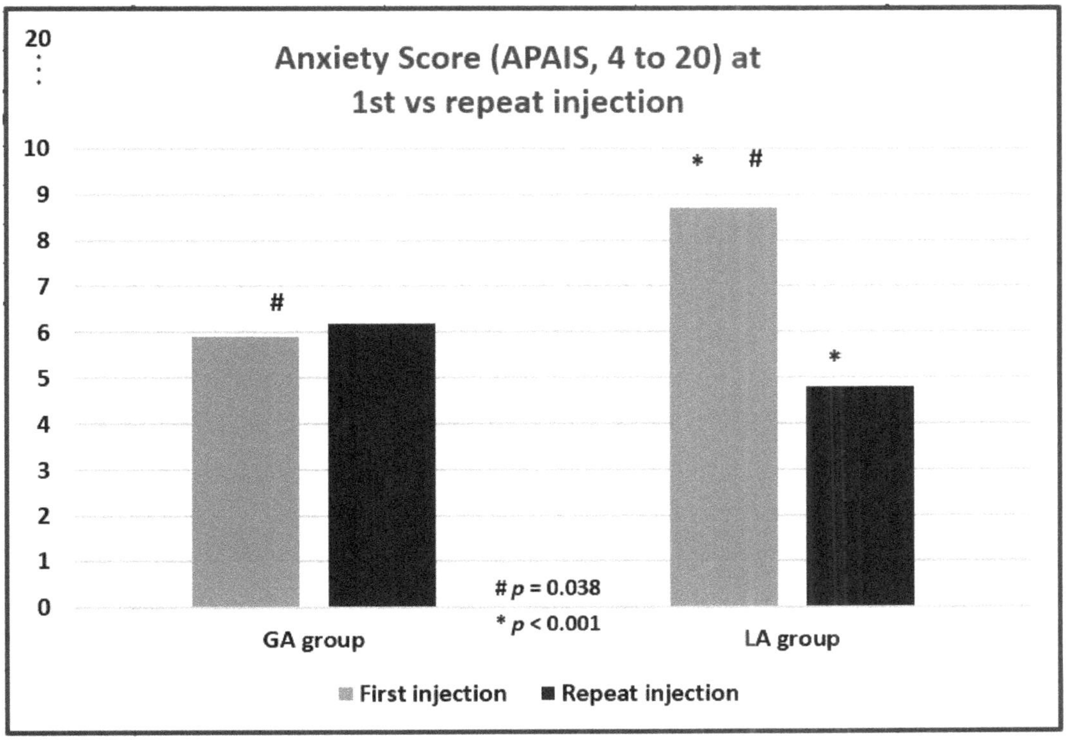

Figure 2. Anxiety Score of the APAIS Questionnaire (Amsterdam Preoperative Anxiety and Information Scale), stratified for first versus repeat injection in the LA and GA groups.

The incontinence questionnaires 4 weeks after the procedure were completed by 55% of the patients ($n = 57$; therapy outcome was no primary variable). All changes in the questionnaires showed highly significant ($p < 0.001$) improvements in symptoms but without significant differences between the LA and GA groups. The changes in this cohort showed a decrease in the Urinary Distress Inventory-6 (UDI-6) score (0–100) from 56.6 to 22.8, in the Incontinence Impact Questionnaire-7 (IIQ-7) score (0–100) from 64.9 to 23.4, in the Symptom Severity Index (SSI) score (0–20) from 11.7 to 5.5, and in the Symptom Impact Index (SII) score (0–12) from 5.1 to 1.5. "Complications from the injection" were not reported by patients in the LA or GA groups. Overall satisfaction with the injection (score 0–10) showed scores of 7.3 ± 3.2 (LA) vs. 8.2 ± 2.6 (GA) ($p = 0.24$). An all-over better bladder/urine control was reported by 86.5% in the LA group and 94.7% in the GA group ($p = 0.77$). Of patients who underwent OnabotA-DI, 84.2% (LA) vs. 94.7% (GA) stated that they would choose this therapy for bladder dysfunction again; the difference was not significant ($p = 0.54$).

Of patients who stated that they had had the procedure performed with both anesthesia methods in the past ($n = 56$), 37 (66%), patients stated that they preferred LA to GA, whereas 19 (34%) preferred GA to LA.

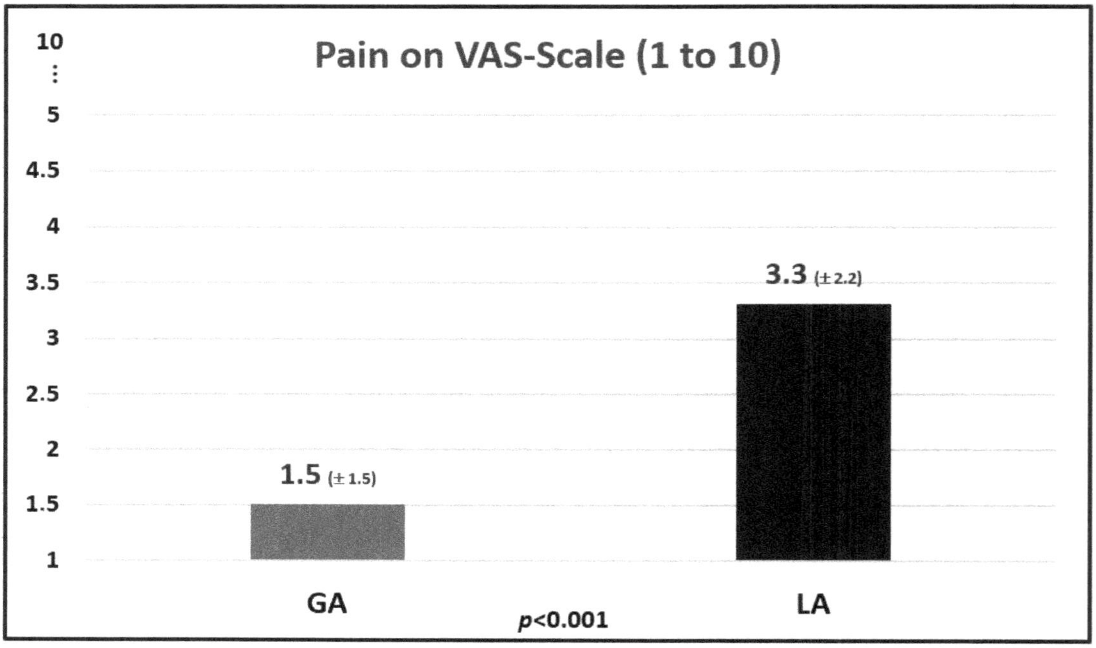

Figure 3. Pain Score on Visual Analog Scale (VAS, can be marked from 1 (no pain) to 10 (worst pain imaginable)) during OnabotA detrusor injection in general anesthesia (GA) and local anesthesia (LA) patients. Values are given in mean (±standard error).

3. Discussion

The OnabotA-DI procedure is well-established in the treatment of hyperactive urinary bladder dysfunction of neurogenic and non-neurogenic origin. The GRACE study was able to report real-world data that documented high patient satisfaction [17].

These results were confirmed in our study using incontinence and quality of life questionnaires 4 weeks after OnabotA-DI. All incontinence scores reflected highly significant improvements. The results did not differ depending on whether the procedure was performed under LA or GA. The results of a satisfaction questionnaire, including questions about complications and choosing this therapy again, also did not differ between groups. As a result, we propose that centers delivering OnabotA-DI can give patients more freedom to choose the type of anesthesia with regard to the expected therapeutic success.

A major obstacle for patients to trust OnabotA-DI is the fear of the procedure, cystoscopy, and especially pain from the injection.

In our study, patients were able to decide for themselves which type of anesthesia they would prefer, LA or GA. Of course, this presents a bias, as GA was primarily chosen by patients who are either very sensitive to pain or have a particular fear of potential pain. To measure this fear before anesthesia or before the procedure, we used the APAIS score. The analysis of the reliability of the APAIS score revealed that the scales were reliable despite their brevity [24] and that the APAIS is also reliable and valid in the German language [25].

In patients who underwent both anesthesia procedures, approximately two-thirds preferred LA and one-third GA. Contrary to popular belief that this procedure is almost always carried out under LA, the frequency with which it is carried out under LA or GA depends on which procedures the patient can choose from. Not all institutions, especially outpatient practices, have an anesthesiologist on staff. In Germany, the procedure under inpatient conditions (where anesthesiologists will always be available) is not reimbursed (with exceptions), so that in the outpatient setting, one has to rely almost exclusively on LA. However, the fear of pain and the different levels of perceived pain should, if possible, be addressed individually by an operating doctor.

An important result of this study is that the Anxiety Score depends on whether the procedure is being carried out for the first time or for a second (or more) time. This finding may contribute to persuading the patient in the primary information discussion to have the procedure carried out under LA, especially since the effort involved in GA is, both for the patient (e.g., fasting before the GA and being accompanied home after the procedure) as well as for the department carrying out the work (e.g., providing an anesthesiologist, operating theater capacity, and costs), much higher.

It is important that the goal must be to allay the fear of significant pain in LA patients, especially before the first injection. The average pain in the LA group in this patient cohort was 3.3 ± 2.2 on the Visual Analogue Scale (VAS), which corresponds to mild to moderate pain. Further effort should be made to make the procedure more comfortable for patients. One possibility would be to allay the patient's fear of "the uncertain procedure". There are successful measures for this in urology. Karalar et al. [26] recently reported a significantly lower feeling of fear and pain in patients during ureteroscopy after presenting the patient with a video of the procedure instead of just verbal communication and information. The group of patients who were presented with an educational video exhibited lower anxiety levels than the patients who only received an educational interview, as reflected by the APAIS scores for anesthesia ($p = 0.02$), surgery ($p < 0.001$), overall ($p < 0.001$), and information needs ($p < 0.001$). An educational video of the OnabotA-DI would be an easy tool to set up in outpatient practice.

Pain-relieving measures also include reducing the number of injection sites while maintaining the same effect, alkalinizing the lidocaine solution [27], reshaping the injection needle [28], and, if necessary, administering further analgesia that has already been applied preoperatively.

4. Conclusions

This study shows significantly different levels of anxiety and pain in patients undergoing OnabotA-DI under LA or GA. Patients' concerns about the perhaps insufficient effect of LA, especially when it is carried out for the first time, should be posed and reflected on by the doctor. In patients who underwent repeated OnabotA-DI, there were no differences in preoperative anxiety levels between LA and GA. However, the different pain levels between LA and GA remained at repeated injections. Since patients prefer LA despite the higher stress level in comparison to GA, future attention must be paid to reducing anxiety before the initial treatment (e.g., through demonstration videos) and to reducing pain through a variety of approaches.

5. Materials and Methods

Patients: Patients who were scheduled for an OnabotA-DI decided for themselves which anesthesia procedure should be used, resulting in two groups: the local anesthesia group (LA) and the general anesthesia group (GA). The indication was for iOAB or nDO, usually due to multiple sclerosis and an expanded disability symptom score of <6, but always with preserved bladder sensitivity and spontaneous bladder emptying (no self-catheterizing patients). In accordance with the requirements of the European guidelines [29], a specific history was carried out including a urine test using urine sediment and a culture to rule out a urinary tract infection or hematuria; an ultrasound with a full bladder to rule out stone disease or a tumor; and a residual urine measurement post micturition. In addition, a vaginal examination was carried out in women to rule out a localized anatomical pathology, such as prolapse, cystocele, or stress incontinence. A digital rectal examination was carried out in men and the Prostate Specific Antigen (PSA) value was measured to rule out prostate cancer.

Measures I: To evaluate the level of anxiety and pain, the APAIS score (4–20; [24,25]) was given during the consultation and the completed form was brought on the day of the operation. To calculate the fear and information score of the APAIS, only completed questionnaires were evaluated.

Procedure: Anticoagulant medication was discontinued in a timely manner according to the information in the package insert; acetylsalicylic acid was continued if necessary. On the day of the injection, the patients remained fasting under GA following the anesthesiologist's instructions. Antibiotic prophylaxis was given preoperatively, usually trimetoprim, which was continued on the evening of the day of the operation and the next morning. Regardless of the anesthesia procedure, the operation was carried out in an outpatient setting. The injection was carried out in the lithotomy position after disinfection and sterile draping. A 21 Char. cystoscope was used with the help of an Albaran (Storz Endoskope, Knittlingen, Germany). According to the study protocol, the injection needle used was a standardized 22-gauge 4 mm needle with a 35 cm long cannula, matching the length of the cystoscope. BotulinumtoxinA was administered in doses of 100, 150, or 200 U of the preparation OnabotulinumtoxinA (Botox®), which was dissolved in 10 mL NaCl. For patients in the GA group, the procedure was carried out immediately after the general anesthetic. In the LA group, the urinary bladder was emptied via a single-use catheter; then, 50 mL lidocaine 2% was instilled, and this lasted for 20 min. The injection scheme included the side walls, posterior wall, bladder base, and trigone. Any minor bleeding that may have occurred was resolved before the procedure was completed. The patients remained in the recovery room of the outpatient clinic for 30–60 min before they were able to leave the practice in the presence of an accompanying person.

Measures II: To record pain, the VAS pain score from 1 to 10 was marked. This VAS score was asked twice in writing to represent intraoperative pain and pain within 24 h after the procedure. The success of the therapy was measured by incontinence questionnaires administered preoperatively and 4 weeks postoperatively (Urinary Distress Inventory UDI-6 (score 0–100): Incontinence Impact Questionnaire IIQ-7 (score 0–100), Symptom Severity Index SSI (score 0–20), and Symptom Impact Index SII (score 0–12)), as well as a general postoperative satisfaction questionnaire, which was aimed, among other things, at pain treatment and the use of painkillers.

The study protocol was approved by the ethics committee of the Universitätsmedizin Berlin (ethics vote number EA4/203/22, ethics committee of the Universitätsmedizin Charité Berlin, Benjamin Franklin Campus).

6. Statistical Tests

Continuous variables such as age were analyzed by calculating the mean, median, standard deviation, and range. Tests for differences between groups were based on either *t*-tests (normally distributed variables) or Wilcoxon's rank-sum test. Categorical variables were characterized by calculating absolute and relative frequencies. Corresponding statistical tests used were Fisher's exact test or the Chi-square test. All analyses were performed with R Core Team (2023). _R: A Language and Environment for Statistical Computing_. R Foundation for Statistical Computing, Vienna, Austria. "R version 4.3.1 (16 June 2023 ucrt)", RStudio Team (2020). RStudio: Integrated Development for R. RStudio, PBC, Boston, MA, USA.

Author Contributions: Conceptualization, H.S.-B. and C.W. (Catarina Weiss); Methodology, H.S.-B., C.W. (Catarina Weiss) and T.S.; Validation, H.S.-B., D.H. and J.N.; Formal Analysis, S.W.; Investigation, H.S.-B. and C.W. (Carsten Waskow); Resources, T.S.; Data Curation, H.S.-B., A.A. and H.B.; Writing—Original Draft Preparation, H.S.-B. and A.A.; Writing—Review and Editing, H.S.-B., H.B., J.N. and B.R.; Visualization, S.W.; Supervision, T.S., J.N. and B.R.; Project Administration, H.S.-B. and K.H. All authors have read and agreed to the published version of the manuscript.

Funding: This research received no external funding.

Institutional Review Board Statement: The study protocol was approved by the ethics committee of the Universitätsmedizin Berlin (ethics vote number EA4/203/22, ethics committee of the Universitätsmedizin Charité Berlin, Benjamin Franklin Campus, approval date: 26 January 2023).

Informed Consent Statement: Informed consent was obtained from all subjects involved in the study.

Data Availability Statement: The raw data supporting the conclusions of this article will be made available by the authors on request.

Acknowledgments: The authors would like to thank Katrin Wolf, Medical Writing, for assistance in completing the manuscript.

Conflicts of Interest: The authors have no conflicts regarding the contents of this study.

References

1. Hu, J.C.; Hsu, L.N.; Lee, W.C.; Chuang, Y.C.; Wang, H.J. Role of Urological Botulinum Toxin-A Injection for Overactive Bladder and Voiding Dysfunction in Patients with Parkinson's Disease or Post-Stroke. *Toxins* **2023**, *15*, 166. [CrossRef]
2. Zulli, A.; Carletti, V.; Mantovani, A.; Cerruto, M.A.; Giacomello, L. Intravesical Botulin Toxin-A Injections for Neurogenic Bladder Dysfunction in Children: Summary Update on Last 10 Years of Research. *Toxins* **2024**, *16*, 339. [CrossRef] [PubMed]
3. Ng, L.G. Botulinum toxin and benign prostatic hyperplasia. *Asian J. Urol.* **2018**, *5*, 33–36. [CrossRef] [PubMed]
4. Chen, J.L.; Kuo, H.C. Clinical application of intravesical botulinum toxin type A for overactive bladder and interstitial cystitis. *Investig. Clin. Urol.* **2020**, *61* (Suppl. S1), S42. [CrossRef] [PubMed]
5. Jiang, Y.H.; Lee, C.L.; Chen, S.F.; Kuo, H.C. Therapeutic Effects of Urethral Sphincter Botulinum Toxin a Injection on Dysfunctional Voiding with Different Videourodynamic Characteristics in Non-Neurogenic Women. *Toxins* **2021**, *13*, 362. [CrossRef] [PubMed]
6. U.S. Food and Drug Administration. FDA Drug Approval Package: Botulinum Toxin Type A. Available online: https://www.accessdata.fda.gov/scripts/cder/daf/index.cfm?event=overview.process&ApplNo=103000 (accessed on 22 September 2024).
7. Apostolidis, A.; Rahnama'i, M.S.; Fry, C.; Dmochowski, R.; Sahai, A. Do we understand how botulinum toxin works and have we optimized the way it is administered to the bladder? ICI-RS 2014. *Neurourol. Urodyn.* **2016**, *35*, 293–298. [CrossRef]
8. Papagiannopoulou, D.; Vardouli, L.; Dimitriadis, F.; Apostolidis, A. Retrograde transport of radiolabelled botulinum neurotoxin type A to the CNS after intradetrusor injection in rats. *BJU Int.* **2016**, *117*, 697–704. [CrossRef]
9. Dmochowski, R.; Chapple, C.; Nitti, V.W.; Chancellor, M.; Everaert, K.; Thompson, C.; Daniell, G.; Zhou, J.; Haag-Molkenteller, C. Efficacy and safety of onabotulinumtoxinA for idiopathic overactive bladder: A double-blind, placebo controlled, randomized, dose ranging trial. *J. Urol.* **2010**, *184*, 2416–2422. [CrossRef]
10. Nitti, V.W.; Dmochowski, R.; Herschorn, S.; Sand, P.; Thompson, C.; Nardo, C.; Yan, X.; Haag-Molkenteller, C.; EMBARK Study Group. OnabotulinumtoxinA for the treatment of patients with overactive bladder and urinary incontinence: Results of a phase 3, randomized, placebo controlled trial. *J. Urol.* **2013**, *189*, 2186–2193. [CrossRef]
11. Nitti, V.W.; Ginsberg, D.; Sievert, K.D.; Sussman, D.; Radomski, S.; Sand, P.; De Ridder, D.; Jenkins, B.; Magyar, A.; Chapple, C.; et al. Durable Efficacy and Safety of Long-Term OnabotulinumtoxinA Treatment in Patients with Overactive Bladder Syndrome: Final Results of a 3.5-Year Study. *J. Urol.* **2016**, *196*, 791–800. [CrossRef]
12. Chapple, C.; Sievert, K.D.; MacDiarmid, S.; Khullar, V.; Radziszewski, P.; Nardo, C.; Thompson, C.; Zhou, J.; Haag-Molkenteller, C. OnabotulinumtoxinA 100 U significantly improves all idiopathic overactive bladder symptoms and quality of life in patients with overactive bladder and urinary incontinence: A randomised, double-blind, placebo-controlled trial. *Eur. Urol.* **2013**, *64*, 249–256. [CrossRef] [PubMed]
13. Cruz, F.; Herschorn, S.; Aliotta, P.; Brin, M.; Thompson, C.; Lam, W.; Daniell, G.; Heesakkers, J.; Haag-Molkenteller, C. Efficacy and safety of onabotulinumtoxinA in patients with urinary incontinence due to neurogenic detrusor overactivity: A randomised, double-blind, placebo-controlled trial. *Eur. Urol.* **2011**, *60*, 742–750. [CrossRef] [PubMed]
14. Kennelly, M.; Dmochowski, R.; Schulte-Baukloh, H.; Ethans, K.; Del Popolo, G.; Moore, C.; Jenkins, B.; Guard, S.; Zheng, Y.; Karsenty, G.; et al. Efficacy and safety of onabotulinumtoxinA therapy are sustained over 4 years of treatment in patients with neurogenic detrusor overactivity: Final results of a long-term extension study. *Neurourol. Urodyn.* **2017**, *36*, 368–375. [CrossRef]
15. Fowler, C.J.; Auerbach, S.; Ginsberg, D.; Hale, D.; Radziszewski, P.; Rechberger, T.; Patel, V.D.; Zhou, J.; Thompson, C.; Kowalski, J.W. OnabotulinumtoxinA improves health-related quality of life in patients with urinary incontinence due to idiopathic overactive bladder: A 36-week, double-blind, placebo-controlled, randomized, dose-ranging trial. *Eur. Urol.* **2012**, *62*, 148–157. [CrossRef]
16. Hamid, R.; Lorenzo-Gomez, M.F.; Schulte-Baukloh, H.; Boroujerdi, A.; Patel, A.; Farrelly, E. OnabotulinumtoxinA is a well tolerated and effective treatment for refractory overactive bladder in real-world practice. *Int. Urogynecol. J.* **2021**, *32*, 65–74. [CrossRef]
17. Farrelly, E.; Hamid, R.; Lorenzo-Gomez, M.F.; Schulte-Baukloh, H.; Yu, J.; Patel, A.; Nelson, M. One treatment with onabotulinumtoxinA relieves symptoms of overactive bladder in patients refractory to one or more oral medications. *Neurourol. Urodyn.* **2023**, *42*, 1203–1213. [CrossRef]
18. Yu, P.H.; Wang, C.C. Adverse Effects of Intravesical OnabotulinumtoxinA Injection in Patients with Idiopathic Overactive Bladder or Neurogenic Detrusor Overactivity: A Systematic Review and Meta-Analysis of Randomized Controlled Studies. *Toxins* **2024**, *16*, 343. [CrossRef]

19. Schulte-Baukloh, H.; Höppner, D.; Hubatsch, M.; Mala, K.; Schlomm, T.; Weinberger, S. Onabotuliumtoxin A detrusor injection: The "real world" of users, the "real world" of patients-Update BOTUROLOGY 2022. *Aktuelle Urol.* **2023**, *54*, 55–60. [CrossRef]
20. DiCarlo-Meacham, A.M.; Dengler, K.L.; Welch, E.K.; Brooks, D.I.; Gruber, D.D.; Osborn, D.J.; Scarlotta, L.; Vaccaro, C.M. Reduced versus standard intradetrusor OnabotulinumtoxinA injections for treatment of overactive bladder. *Neurourol. Urodyn.* **2023**, *42*, 366–374. [CrossRef]
21. Chang, E.S.; Ringel, N.; Woodburn, K.L.; Tanner, J.P.; Bassaly, R.; Greene, K.; Wyman, A.; Iglesia, C. Postprocedural Pain Associated With 5 Versus 20 Intradetrusor Injections of onabotulinumtoxinA for Treatment of Overactive Bladder: A Multicenter Randomized Clinical Trial. *Urogynecology* **2022**, *28*, 518–525. [CrossRef]
22. Pereira ESilva, R.; Ponte, C.; Lopes, F.; Palma Dos Reis, J. Alkalinized lidocaine solution as a first-line local anesthesia protocol for intradetrusor injection of onabotulinum toxin A: Results from a double-blinded randomized controlled trial. *Neurourol. Urodyn.* **2020**, *39*, 2471–2479. [CrossRef] [PubMed]
23. Schurch, B.; Reitz, A.; Tenti, G. Electromotive drug administration of lidocaine to anesthetize the bladder before botulinum-A toxin injections into the detrusor. *Spinal Cord* **2004**, *42*, 338–341. [CrossRef] [PubMed]
24. Moerman, N.; van Dam, F.S.; Muller, M.J.; Oosting, H. The Amsterdam Preoperative Anxiety and Information Scale (APAIS). *Anesth. Analg.* **1996**, *82*, 445–451. [CrossRef] [PubMed]
25. Berth, H.; Petrowski, K.; Balck, F. The Amsterdam Preoperative Anxiety and Information Scale (APAIS)-the first trial of a German version. *Psychosoc. Med.* **2007**, *4*, Doc01. [PubMed] [PubMed Central]
26. Karalar, M.; Demirbas, A.; Gercek, O.; Topal, K.; Keles, I. Impact of Preoperative Video-Based Education on Anxiety Levels in Patients with Renal Stones Scheduled for Flexible Ureteroscopic Lithotripsy: A Comparative Study Using APAIS and STAI. *Med. Sci. Monit.* **2023**, *29*, e941351-1. [CrossRef]
27. Faure Walker, N.; Macpherson, F.; Tasleem, A.; Rampal, T. Interventions to improve tolerability of local anesthetic intradetrusor Botulinum toxin injections: A systematic review. *Neurourol. Urodyn.* **2023**, *42*, 23–32. [CrossRef]
28. Hameed, F.; Anwaar, A.; Karamat, R.I.; Anwar, M. Improving intravesical botulinum toxin-A injection technique: Reshaping the needle may benefit more. *Investig. Clin. Urol.* **2024**, *65*, 522–523. [CrossRef]
29. Nambiar, A.K.; Arlandis, S.; Bø, K.; Cobussen-Boekhorst, H.; Costantini, E.; de Heide, M.; Farag, F.; Groen, J.; Karavitakis, M.; Lapitan, M.C.; et al. European Association of Urology Guidelines on the Diagnosis and Management of Female Non-neurogenic Lower Urinary Tract Symptoms. Part 1: Diagnostics, Overactive Bladder, Stress Urinary Incontinence, and Mixed Urinary Incontinence. *Eur. Urol.* **2022**, *82*, 49–59. [CrossRef]

toxins

Perspective

Expert Opinions on Best Practices for Overactive Bladder Management with onabotulinumtoxinA

Karyn S. Eilber [1,*], Benjamin M. Brucker [2], Andrea Pezzella [3], Vincent Lucente [4,5,6], Kevin Benson [7] and Michael J. Kennelly [8]

1 Department of Urology, Cedars-Sinai Medical Center, Los Angeles, CA 90211, USA
2 Departments of Urology and Obstetrics and Gynecology, New York University Langone Health, New York, NY 10016, USA
3 Southern Urogynecology Wellness and Aesthetics, West Columbia, SC 29169, USA
4 Axia Women's Health, The Institute for Female Pelvic Medicine & Reconstructive Surgery, FPM Urogynecology Center, Allentown, PA 18103, USA
5 Division of Gynecology, Section of Urogynecology, St. Luke's University Health Network, Bethlehem, PA 18015, USA
6 Department of Obstetrics and Gynecology, Lewis Katz School of Medicine at Temple University, Philadelphia, PA 19140, USA
7 Department of Obstetrics and Gynecology, Division of Urogynecology and Pelvic Surgery, Sanford University of South Dakota Medical Center and Hospital, Sioux Falls, SD 57105, USA
8 Department of Urology, Atrium Health Wake Forest University School of Medicine, Carolinas Medical Center, Charlotte, NC 28203, USA
* Correspondence: karyn.eilber@cshs.org

Abstract

OnabotulinumtoxinA is an FDA-approved treatment for adults with overactive bladder (OAB) who have an inadequate response to, or are intolerant of, oral pharmacotherapies including anticholinergics or beta-3 agonists. However, procedural practices of onabotulinumtoxinA intradetrusor injection vary among practitioners and can affect patient experience. To address this, a panel of six high-volume intravesical onabotulinumtoxinA providers with 100 years of combined experience convened to discuss the best office practices when treating patients with OAB. These key best practices include counseling patients on available OAB therapies, including onabotulinumtoxinA, at the initial consultation in accordance with established AUA and SUFU guidelines in a way that is easily understood. An office setting is preferred over a hospital or surgery center when performing the procedure. Staff involvement, from scheduling to post-procedure, is essential for establishing the relationships necessary to optimize patient experience and encourage compliance and retreatment. Experts generally recommend using a viscous lidocaine bladder instillation for an anesthetic 15 min prior to the reconstitution of onabotulinumtoxinA with 5 to 10 mL of normal saline. A range of one to 20 injection sites is acceptable, with a smaller number preferred. Starting in the lower bladder, experts recommend using a slower speed of injection to improve distribution and decrease patient discomfort. Subsequent treatments should be regularly scheduled at six-month intervals with the option of re-treating earlier if symptoms return, but no sooner than 12 weeks. For office intravesical onabotulinumtoxinA procedures, optimization of the patient experience by the physician and their staff, starting with the initial visit through the post-treatment follow-up, is key to long-term patient compliance.

Keywords: overactive bladder; onabotulinumtoxinA; urge incontinence; botox; procedure considerations; minimally invasive therapy

Key Contribution: After a decade since approval, clear recommendations for onabotA use in overactive bladder are lacking. These best practices, based on opinions from experts, provide additional guidance for clinical practice.

1. Introduction

Overactive bladder (OAB) is defined by the International Continence Society as urinary urgency usually accompanied by frequency and nocturia, with or without urge urinary incontinence [1]. OAB is a chronic condition that impacts patients' quality of life and requires long-term management. The available treatment options for the treatment of OAB include non-invasive (mainly behavioral) therapies, oral pharmacotherapy, minimally invasive intravesical therapy, tibial or sacral neuromodulation, and surgical intervention (bladder augmentation). The American Urological Association (AUA) and the Society of Urodynamics, Female Pelvic Medicine and Urogenital Reconstruction (SUFU) emphasize the importance of shared decision-making to select the best therapy or therapies based on the patient's needs, desires, and tolerance of side effects over the concept of "step therapy" [2].

OnabotulinumtoxinA (onabotA) is an FDA-approved, minimally invasive option for the treatment of adult patients with OAB and symptoms of urge urinary incontinence, urgency, and frequency [3]. The AUA guidelines recommend onabotA in patients who have failed an oral pharmacotherapy or for those who are unable or unwilling to undertake behavioral or pharmacological treatments. Studies have demonstrated that onabotA is safe and effective over repeated treatments that are typically readministered between 4 and 7.6 months [4–6].

While the clinical trials performed for the FDA approval of onabotA provide a framework for the procedure, individual practices vary [7]. Similar rates of clinical efficacy and adverse events have been reported for different injection paradigms, without clear recommendations [8–10]. Multiple non-inferior bladder analgesic options are available for procedural pain control [11], and there are few evidence-based recommendations regarding peri-procedural antibiotic prophylaxis surrounding onabotA treatment to reduce the risk of procedure-related urinary tract infection (UTI) [12]. While many clinicians embrace practice variability, this same variability may deter many practitioners from offering onabotA to their OAB patients. As a result, an expert panel including urologists and urogynecologists with high office volumes (10 to 20 intravesical onabotA patients per week) and with 100 years of combined experience convened to discuss their personal experiences and current research through moderator-led questions on focused topics in an effort to provide additional guidance for clinical practice. The experts were selected based on their credentials, years of experience, involvement in research, and reputations as experts amongst their peers. This paper summarizes the discussion from this group of six experts who routinely use onabotA to treat adults with OAB and describes best practices based on their opinions. The experts reviewed when and how to introduce onabotA to patients, effective approaches for the procedure day, and post-procedural care to allow for a positive treatment experience and improve long-term compliance.

2. Pre-Procedural Considerations

2.1. Introducing the Care Pathway

By the time a patient visits a specialist, they have typically tried one or more oral agent(s) that have been prescribed by another provider. After assessing and confirming the diagnosis of OAB, the health care professional (a physician or advanced care practitioner such as a physician assistant or nurse practitioner) should spend time introducing the OAB care options. The non-invasive (behavioral modification), pharmacologic, and minimally invasive therapies as recommended by the AUA/SUFU OAB guidelines should be discussed [2]. Patients and clinicians should talk openly about medication side effects, the potential risks of the various therapies, and issues such as accessibility and cost for patients in the US. It is important to start the conversation on the available therapies, including minimally invasive options such as onabotA, at the initial visit so that the patient is aware of the many therapeutic options for OAB to provide hope for finding a successful treatment [13]. Introducing onabotA early allows for patients' familiarity with this treatment option and prepares them to more readily discuss it—if and when the time comes. It should be reinforced that regardless of the treatment a patient chooses, behavioral modification and fluid restriction are always important.

When initially explaining minimally invasive therapies, provide patients with key points and avoid making the discussion too complicated. The goal is to introduce the treatment options while keeping the explanations simple in order to give patients a sense of hope and a reason to return. For example, explain that there are effective options beyond diet and behavioral changes that, in some cases, may work more effectively than oral medications. Of the available minimally invasive therapies and taking into consideration patients' preferences along with the therapy's efficacy, ease of administration, mechanism of action, concomitant conditions, and cost, the experts view onabotA as a simple way to provide effective treatment for their patients. OnabotA is also a popular option with patients: when patients were asked to rank their preferences of minimally invasive therapies after being provided with the risks and benefits of each option, most chose onabotA as their first choice based on its long-term efficacy [14].

When introducing onabotA, highlight the therapy's efficacy to give patients hope and expectations of success. In two Phase 3 clinical trials, onabotA significantly decreased the daily frequency of urinary incontinence episodes and improved all other overactive bladder symptoms compared to placebo [4,15]. Up to 31% of patients became completely continent, and the patient health-related quality of life was significantly improved [4,6,15]. Empower the patient not to settle—OAB is common, but it is not merely a normal part of aging [2]. Discussing the patient's quality of life is important, especially for those who have a difficult time making treatment decisions. Focus on lifestyle improvements: Are they living their best possible life? There is always an opportunity for improvement. Experts typically set a realistic expectation of relieving patients' symptoms by at least 75%, with the goal of becoming symptom-free. For patients in the US, explain that onabotA is typically covered by most insurance plans and that additional assistance can be provided for commercial insurance patients.

Move on to how it is administered, while using non-technical phrases that are easily understood, such as "it is placed in your bladder" [3]. When counseling on the risk of post-procedure incomplete bladder emptying, make sure to use patient-friendly language, such as "Nearly all patients could still urinate when they needed to, but some patients may not be able to fully empty their bladder" [3,16]. In the rare case of a patient needing to catheterize, explain that they do not need to have a "bag," and describe self-management using clean intermittent catheterization (CIC) as an alternative way to drain the bladder with a small tube about the size of a coffee stirrer. Educate the patient that retreatment is usually every six months to prevent symptoms from returning, but it can be flexible depending on their schedule [3–5]. Most importantly, assure them that the provider and the staff at the practice will be with them through the entire treatment process to provide counsel at every step of the way. It is a partnership and not a journey for the patient alone. If the patient is not satisfied with onabotA or if they decide to move on to something else, other minimally invasive treatments can be considered as an alternative [2].

2.2. Shared Decision-Making: Determining Whether OnabotA Is the Right Therapy for the Patient

The patient's preferences and logistical considerations can be critical to the treatment choice [2]. Non-medical factors often play a role in making recommendations for the patient. The provider should pose questions to understand their concerns, which may rule out alternative minimally invasive options such as neuromodulation: What is their lifestyle like? Is it feasible to return weekly for 12 weeks and then monthly for percutaneous tibial nerve stimulation (PTNS)? Are they technologically savvy enough to interact with a neuromodulation device that is implanted? How do they feel about a procedure that can require sedation or anesthesia? Are they willing to undergo repeated office procedures? OnabotA is a good option for patients unwilling to have minimally invasive surgery or staged treatment phases, which often have lifestyle restrictions. Many patients also tend to like that onabotA is not permanent. OnabotA should be an obvious choice for patients who absolutely do not want surgery, are not surgical candidates, and/or cannot return regularly for the maintenance of a neuromodulation device.

OnabotA is contraindicated in patients who have an active urinary tract infection, a known allergy to botulinum toxin or its components, or a post-void residual (PVR) over 200 mL who are not routinely performing CIC [3]. There are certain patient populations that may require special considerations, such as those who may be at a higher risk for incomplete bladder emptying and who are not performing CIC at baseline, including patients with diabetes or neurogenic bladder, those over 70 years old, and male patients with benign prostatic hyperplasia [3,17–19]. Body dystocia, arthritis, or any other physical disability resulting in the patient's inability to physically catheterize should also be taken into consideration [3,4]. A summary of the benefits, potential side effects, and contraindications is provided in Table 1.

Table 1. Benefits, potential side effects, and contraindications of onabotA for OAB.

Benefits
• Most patients have at least 75% relief of symptoms • Up to 31% of patients became completely continent in clinical trials • Long-term safety and efficacy • Significant improvements in QOL • Reversible • Infrequent (average twice yearly) office treatments
Potential Side Effects
• UTI • Temporary inability to void • Dysuria • Increased residual urine volume
Absolute Contraindications
• PVR > 200 mL in those not routinely performing CIC • Active UTI • Hypersensitivity to botulinum toxins or any of the components in the formulation

CIC = clean intermittent catheterization; OAB = overactive bladder; PVR = post-void residual; QOL = quality of life; UTI = urinary tract infection.

Using a holistic approach (Box 1), the provider should carefully assess each individual situation, be able to clearly explain why the therapy is being recommended, and use shared decision-making to determine what is best for the patient [2]. Most patients have already tried and failed other OAB treatments (including multiple medications) and are looking to you for guidance.

Box 1. A holistic approach to prescribing treatments for OAB.

A holistic approach to prescribing treatments for OAB considers not only the medical condition but also the patient's unique circumstances [2]. Consider the patient's viewpoint when evaluating the options, given their unique circumstances, including psychosocial, economic, social support, and educational factors.Psychosocial Factors.

- Patient Preferences: Involve patients in decision-making when discussing treatment options.
- Cultural Beliefs: Cultural context may affect acceptance of and/or adherence to certain therapies.
- Social Support: Consider the patient's support system and ability to manage medications and appointments.

Economic Factors for US Patients

- Affordability: Assess whether the patient can afford the prescribed medication.
- Insurance Coverage: Check whether the drug is covered by the patient's insurance plan.

Practical Considerations

- Route of Administration: Choose an appropriate form (oral, injectable, topical).
- Frequency: Consider dosing frequency and convenience for the patient.
- Storage: Ensure patients can store and handle the medication properly.

Adherence and Education

- Patient Education: Provide clear instructions, potential side effects, and warnings.
- Monitoring: Regularly assess treatment effectiveness and address any issues.

The experts have felt that onabotA is their "go-to," as it does very well with the holistic approach. taking all of these factors into account.

2.3. Where Should the Procedure Take Place?

OnabotA procedures can be performed in the office, an ambulatory surgery center, or a hospital surgery suite; however, the experts feel that for the optimal patient acceptability of long-term onabotA treatment, the procedures should be performed in the office [20]. Establishing a well-run, office-based onabotA practice ensures efficiency for both patients and providers. It considers the patient's perspective regarding cost, time management, and adherence. As the actual time spent by the physician on the onabotA injection is typically only a few minutes, time can be lost by traveling to another location and/or by surgical delays. For the provider, best practices are easier to tailor in an office setting and makes post-procedural follow-up more practical.

For a minority of patients, there may be exceptions or mitigating circumstances that make a location other than the office preferable. Office procedures may be impractical for some patients due to their pain intolerance or inability to position themselves without significant pain or because of a physical disability. Using a facility that offers sedation may be more desirable for patients who have medically complicated situations or those with OAB caused by a neurological condition. Moreover, not all providers can perform the procedure in the office; for example, they may lack equipment such as cystoscopes. The use of an ambulatory surgery center or hospital operating room not only accommodates these situations but also offers providers who are new to injecting onabotA the opportunity to build this skill set. Performing the first few onabotA procedures with sedation is a great way to gain experience and help transition the provider to the office setting.

2.4. Logistics of Practice: Are You Set Up for Success?

The logistics of practice are essential for providers who are just starting to use onabotA. Regarding access, is your office set up to accommodate a certain volume of patients in a timely manner? Can your office or procedure room handle repeat procedures? Regarding the equipment and setup, consider the number of cystoscopes available. Single-use, disposable cystoscopes can be an effective, safe, and affordable alternative to reusable scopes to accommodate a high volume of patients [21,22]. Single-use cystoscopes also reduce the need for the staff to process equipment or to delay or limit procedures based on availability. Regarding onabotA inventory, consider the financial and storage capacities of your practice. Assess the need for a buy-and-bill process and the ability to properly store onabotA, which also extends to inventory management and expiration date tracking.

3. Day of Procedure Considerations

3.1. Emphasizing the Patient Experience

The experts emphasize that the force driving the overall success of repeat treatments is the patient's experience. The atmosphere should be comfortable and appealing from the moment the patient walks into the office to the conclusion of the procedure. There are several considerations that can help with patients' comfort and anxiety, such as dimming the lights, letting the patient choose the music, and offering a blanket and/or aromatherapy. A recent study on the use of aromatherapy and music during magnetic resonance imaging procedures suggested these could reduce anxiety and improve patients' comfort [23]. Anxiety can also be reduced by keeping items used for the procedure, such as the cystoscope, out of the patient's view. Distracting the patient with ongoing dialogue is also useful [24]. Encourage patients to keep their eyes open during the procedure, as it requires greater central nervous system processing of vision, which can decrease pain perception [25]. It may be beneficial to encourage patients to take an over-the-counter oral analgesic or nonsteroidal anti-inflammatory medication upon leaving their residence for the procedure.

Be consistent in your procedural flow, as patients will become used to the process and have proper expectations. Having a favorable environment and a relaxed patient also benefits the medical assistants. Soliciting patients' feedback is a great way to keep finding new ideas for process improvements and to incorporate patients' preferences for repeat visits. Patients appreciate when providers make an obvious effort to ensure their comfort. They value the personal touches. Interpersonal interactions are important, and continuity with regard to staff is key. According to the experts, they estimate that approximately 70% of their patients come back for retreatment based on a positive experience with the staff, which may be challenging for practices that have high turnover or different staff members on irregular schedules. When consistency in the staff is not possible, additional staff training or referencing documented patient feedback for procedural preferences may be an alternative. Patients like to feel that the staff are their friends and that they can see a familiar face at each visit. Demonstrated care for patients' wellbeing and comfort by the front desk staff and schedulers can help with the feeling that appointments are transactional. For example, having the same nurses perform the follow-up and the two-week post-procedure check-in not only allows the staff to assess how the patients are doing but also enables the patient to experience a true connection. These interpersonal relationships add to the sense of lifestyle improvement. When you get to know the patient, the resulting trust and care they feel play a major role in giving them a reason to return for all procedures in your office, not just for the onabotA treatments.

Regarding staff retention, when staff members feel connected, they are also more likely to stay. In a larger organization, a sense of ownership by the staff members can become lost if there is no clear direction on individual responsibility. Physicians have a true leadership responsibility in this area, taking the reins and outlining the expectations. These can be verbalized or written down. While care maps are frequently utilized for patients, they are also needed for the staff. How does your staff fit into the overall process? Make their roles clear. During staff training or when onboarding new staff members, emphasize the focus on the patient experience over efficiency. The staff truly shapes the experience, so encourage them to have a sense of ownership and make them feel empowered. Allow your staff to take control of setting up the procedure room, informing patients about antibiotics, and being there to hold their hands during the procedure. The physician may be the injector providing the treatment, but it is the staff that sustains the positive, service-based experience.

3.2. Obtaining Consent

In the US, state and local requirements may vary, but patient consent should be obtained before each procedure. After the original consent form is signed, some experts suggest obtaining an abbreviated consent by having patients re-initial and date the original consent on each subsequent visit. Others prefer to require renewed consent with each round of onabotA and a review of the risks and benefits, which allows patients to have their questions answered prior to the procedure. This step should be individualized to satisfy the requirements and balanced with efficiency to ensure that providers have sufficient time to maximize their productivity.

3.3. Pre-Procedure Urinalysis

The expert opinions vary on the use of pre-procedure urinalysis (UA), and it is ultimately left to the discretion of the clinician. Performing a UA prior to the procedure day when a patient has no acute urinary tract infection (UTI) complaints can lead to an unnecessary cancellation if there are UA findings but the patient is asymptomatic. However, for some clinicians, the presence of asymptomatic bacteriuria may deserve further discussion and/or intervention. Some experts recommend performing a dipstick test on the day of the procedure, but this could potentially lead to aborted procedures, so experts who recommend this also prescribe pre-procedure antibiotics (see next section). Some suggest following the AUA guidelines for asymptomatic bacteriuria screening [26]. Others simply check whether the patient is symptomatic by asking, "Do you have burning with urination?" Symptoms suggestive of a UTI would prompt a UA before the procedure. Some experts who do not perform a UA will delay reconstituting onabotA until they have visualized the bladder by cystoscopy and will only proceed if the bladder mucosa has a normal appearance, which can rule out a local inflammation suggestive of an active infection. The experts agree that the procedure must be cancelled if there is an active infection.

3.4. Prophylactic Periprocedural Antibiotics

The experts agree that some form of a prophylactic antibiotic may be beneficial to ensure the patient does not arrive on the procedure day with a UTI, resulting in an aborted procedure, or that a subclinical UTI does not progress after the procedure is performed. The choice of an antibiotic can be made based on the patient's allergies and the AUA guideline for a cystourethroscopy with manipulation that recommends a single dose of either a fluoroquinolone, trimethoprim-sulfamethoxazole, aminoglycoside, first- or second-generation cephalosporin, or amoxicillin-clavulanate [26]. However, caution is warranted for the concomitant use of onabotA and aminoglycosides [3]. One expert recommends giving a 3-day course of antibiotics starting on the day before the procedure, while others administer an oral antibiotic right before or immediately after the procedure as one dose with success. This single dose is convenient for patients, saving them a trip to the pharmacy. For patients with a history of recurrent UTIs, or for those traveling a greater distance who could be impacted by cancellation/rescheduling, antibiotics could be considered at least one day before the procedure. Antibiotic stewardship should be considered, especially in older patients. Taken together, there is some variability in the timing of the prophylactic antibiotic course used by the experts based on the individual patient circumstances since the data varies on whether antibiotic use, regimen, and route impact the post-procedure UTI rates [27].

3.5. Discontinuation of Anticoagulants and Antiplatelets

Anticoagulants and antiplatelets may be discontinued prior to the onabotA procedure, but it is not required [28]. The experts agree that the use of smaller gauge needles and the proper direct visualization of the blood vessels allow for safe procedures when patients are on blood thinners. Ultimately, it is left to the discretion of the provider and the consideration of the bleeding risk.

3.6. Local Analgesia or Anesthesia for the OnabotulinumtoxinA Procedure

Oral phenazopyridine may be administered the night before and the morning of the procedure, as a substitute or in addition to topical intravesical lidocaine to enhance patient comfort [11]. Patients using phenazopyridine should be instructed to anticipate orange urine that may stain clothing. Experts recommend using a viscous lidocaine bladder instillation at least 15 min before the onabotA procedure. One expert recommends pre-packaging supplies ahead of time and having everything pre-mixed to allow for the lidocaine instillation as quickly as possible after the initial intake. During the instillation dwell time, vitals can be taken, the UA may be processed if a sample was taken, and a patient preference sheet can be completed to recreate or improve the experience for the next appointment. The experts proceed with the onabotA procedures with the lidocaine remaining in the bladder to improve the procedure's overall efficiency and based on a lack of evidence to the contrary.

3.7. Type of Cystoscope

Both rigid and flexible cystoscopes are appropriate for use in onabotA procedures, with different advantages for each [4,29]. The flexible cystoscope is a two-person procedure, while the rigid cystoscope is a one-person procedure. With a rigid cystoscope, the medical assistant can be focused on ensuring patient comfort, such as by holding the patient's hand while having an engaging conversation. If an assistant is needed for the injection process, seamless communication is required for the proper injection timing. If you have a new medical assistant or other personnel requiring verbal communication, set the expectation with the patient ahead of time so that they are comfortable with the verbal exchange.

3.8. Injection Paradigms: Dose, Location, Volume, and Number of Injection Sites

Over the years, many injection paradigms have been explored. The onabotA United States Prescribing Information (USPI) details a 20-injection site paradigm using a total dose of 100 Units (U) as 0.5 mL (5 U) injections across 20 sites into the detrusor [3]. The Phase 4 LO-BOT study evaluated an alternative injection paradigm using 100 U of onabotA reconstituted with 5 mL of normal saline and administered as 10 injections of 0.5 mL—two in the trigone and eight distributed evenly across the posterior wall of the bladder around the trigonal area [30]. The use of this paradigm resulted in improved treatment benefits over placebo with a low incidence of incomplete bladder emptying requiring CIC.

The optimal number of injections maximizes the distribution while minimizing the number of injection sites. The experts recommend a range from one to 20 injection sites based on experience and available data, balancing the number of injections with efficacy and patients' comfort [3,10,30–32]. Most of the experts recommend fewer injections while balancing the fact that onabotA must be adequately taken up by the peripheral nerve terminals. The expert panel agrees that the number and location of injections can be customized for each patient. Based on a meta-analysis, trigonal-involved onabotA injections were more effective compared with trigone-sparing injections [33], likely due to the dense innervation of the trigone [34]. Ultimately, the decision should be made at the time of the injection based on the patient's comfort and technical considerations such as the patient's anatomy and the ease of reaching all of the intended injection sites.

When performing a minimal injection paradigm, the experts recommend initiating the first dose of onabotA at 100 U, with a reconstitution volume of 5 to 10 mL and using 0.5 to 5.0 mL per injection site, based on diffusion [3,35]. A dose titration up to 200 U may be considered in patients who have an inadequate response and minimal side effects [2]. When patients return, information on symptomatology can be correlated with the dose, volume, and number of injections, and adjustments can be made accordingly. This will allow for the reevaluation of optimal diffusion, with the objective of reaching more presynaptic nerve terminals.

3.9. Depth and Rate of Injections

The experts agree that the depth or plane of injection is important for the efficient lateral distribution of onabotA, especially when attempting to use fewer injection sites. The afferent nerves are located in the superficial suburothelium and are appropriate to target for OAB dry (without urge incontinence) [36], while the efferent nerves are in the deeper detrusor section of the urothelium and are appropriate for OAB wet (with urge incontinence) [37]. Adding a drop of dye such as sodium fluorescein is an off-label suggestion to optimize the technique, and it may help visualize the outline of the injection and enable a better determination of the correct injection depth that is not too superficial [38]. A "groundswell" should be visible with minimal pressure. Adjust the needle if necessary to maintain an optimal depth, as too superficial of an injection results in a bleb [29], which is not desirable. The rate of infiltration is also an important consideration; the slower the rate, the greater the dispersion, with less pain experienced. Force should never be used since it generates more pressure. A slower infiltration also allows for easier adjustments if the needle is at the wrong depth, as evidenced by a loss of the onabotA out of the injection site and/or the development of a bleb.

4. Post-Treatment Considerations

4.1. Management of Adverse Events

Incomplete bladder emptying leading to an elevated PVR has been observed following onabotA treatment, and in some cases, this may require temporary treatment using CIC [3, 17]. Most of the experts recommend only performing a PVR test once, two weeks after the initial treatment. A post-procedure PVR after subsequent treatments is considered generally unnecessary unless the patient has had a dose increase, if there is a lack of improvement in OAB symptoms following the procedure, or if the patient had a significantly elevated PVR (generally with symptoms of incomplete emptying) after their first treatment. In consideration of the age-based risk stratification for the incidence and duration of post-procedural CIC [39], some of the experts tend to be more liberal with younger patients but more conservative with older patients when determining the need for a post-procedural PVR. The experts agree that patients with a PVR >250 mL do not necessarily need to perform CIC, but the ultimate decision can be made based on the patient's symptoms and the overall clinical picture [16].

The onset of onabotA is approximately 1–2 weeks [40]; therefore, any OAB medications can be discontinued after one week of the procedure with a minimal risk of retention. However, patients should be instructed to discontinue them sooner if voiding difficulty ensues.

4.2. Retreatment

Make a conscious effort to set up follow-up appointments. The office staff can help navigate the patient back for additional treatments. Most experts agree that patients should be proactively scheduled for their next procedure before leaving the office rather than waiting until they have symptoms to avoid a significant delay for subsequent procedures and/or the return of symptoms. There is variability in the duration of patients' responses; for some, symptoms may return in four months, and for others, they do not return for eight months to a year [3–6]. Regardless of when symptoms return, most of the experts schedule a follow-up treatment six months following the first procedure to avoid having time without effective therapy. Setting up retreatment visits every six months is common practice, and appointments can be rescheduled earlier if symptoms return sooner. Six months is consistent with the retreatment paradigms of the pivotal onabotA clinical trials and the open label extension studies [3–5,41]. Patients who are traveling or have an upcoming special event to attend may receive reinjections earlier, but no sooner than 12 weeks after their last procedure [3].

5. Final Thoughts

While onabotA was approved by the FDA in 2013 for the treatment of adults with OAB, procedural practices still vary among practitioners, and clinicians often seek advice on how to appropriately manage patients with OAB using onabotA. Table 2 summarizes the recommendations of an expert panel of providers with 100 years of combined intravesical onabotA experience in an effort to provide additional guidance and recommendations for clinical practice.

Table 2. Summary of expert recommendations.

Category	Recommendations
Pre-procedural considerations	• Discuss OAB care pathway using simple language • Perform the onabotA procedure in an office, not a hospital • Ensure practice is set up for success
Day of procedure considerations	• Emphasize patient experience • Check for UTI symptoms, perform UA if needed • Use prophylactic antibiotics • Use lidocaine gel 15 min before procedure • Reconstitute 100 U vial with 5 to 10 mL • 1 to 20 injection sites, balance comfort and diffusion • Slow instillation reduces pain
Post-procedural considerations	• Perform 2-week PVR once after initial treatment unless dose is increased • Proactively schedule next procedure every 6 months • Move up appointments if symptoms return sooner

OAB = overactive bladder; PVR = post-void residual; U = units; UA = urinalysis; UTI = urinary tract infection.

Author Contributions: All authors were responsible for conceptualization, original draft preparation, reviewing, and editing. All authors have read and agreed to the published version of the manuscript.

Funding: AbbVie provided organizational and logistical support for the expert consensus and funded independent medical writing support according to the Good Publication Practice guideline.

Institutional Review Board Statement: This panel was deemed exempt from Institutional Review Board review.

Data Availability Statement: No new data were created or analyzed in this study. Data sharing is not applicable to this article.

Acknowledgments: Medical writing/editorial assistance was provided by Jaime S. Horton of CD Chunn & Associates.

Conflicts of Interest: A.P.: Consultant for AbbVie and Neuspera, Investigator for Axonics; B M.B.: Speaker, Advisor, and/or Investigator for AbbVie, Axonics, Sumitomo Pharma, Provepharma, and Watkins Conti Medtronic. Education grant recipient of Medtronic and Axonics; K.B.: Consultant for AbbVie, Boston Scientific, and Medtronic; K.S.E.: Consultant for AbbVie and Boston Scientific, Investigator for Abbvie and Coloplast; M.J.K.: Advisory Board and/or Grant/Research support from AbbVie, Axonics, Becton Dickinson, Coloplast, Cook Myosite, Medtronic, SpineX, and Urovant; V.L.: Speaker, Consultant, and Investigator for AbbVie.

References

1. Abrams, P.; Cardozo, L.; Fall, M.; Griffiths, D.; Rosier, P.; Ulmsten, U.; Van Kerrebroeck, P.; Victor, A.; Wein, A. The standardisation of terminology in lower urinary tract function: Report from the standardisation sub-committee of the international continence society. *Urology* **2003**, *61*, 37–49. [CrossRef] [PubMed]
2. Cameron, A.P.; Chung, D.E.; Dielubanza, E.J.; Enemchukwu, E.; Ginsberg, D.A.; Helfand, B.T.; Linder, B.J.; Reynolds, W.S.; Rovner, E.S.; Souter, L.; et al. The aua/sufu guideline on the diagnosis and treatment of idiopathic overactive bladder. *J. Urol.* **2024**, *212*, 11–20. [CrossRef]
3. Abbvie. Botox [Package Insert]. U.S. Food and Drug Administration Website. Revised August 2023. Available online: https://www.accessdata.fda.gov/drugsatfda_docs/label/2023/103000orig1s5325correctedlbl.pdf (accessed on 21 June 2024).
4. Nitti, V.W.; Dmochowski, R.; Herschorn, S.; Sand, P.; Thompson, C.; Nardo, C.; Yan, X.; Haag-Molkenteller, C. Onabotulinumtoxina for the treatment of patients with overactive bladder and urinary incontinence: Results of a phase 3, randomized, placebo controlled trial. *J. Urol.* **2013**, *189*, 2186–2193. [CrossRef]
5. Nitti, V.W.; Ginsberg, D.; Sievert, K.D.; Sussman, D.; Radomski, S.; Sand, P.; De Ridder, D.; Jenkins, B.; Magyar, A.; Chapple, C. Durable efficacy and safety of long-term onabotulinumtoxina treatment in patients with overactive bladder syndrome: Final results of a 3.5-year study. *J. Urol.* **2016**, *196*, 791–800. [CrossRef]
6. Chapple, C.; Sievert, K.D.; MacDiarmid, S.; Khullar, V.; Radziszewski, P.; Nardo, C.; Thompson, C.; Zhou, J.; Haag-Molkenteller, C. Onabotulinumtoxina 100 u significantly improves all idiopathic overactive bladder symptoms and quality of life in patients with overactive bladder and urinary incontinence: A randomised, double-blind, placebo-controlled trial. *Eur. Urol.* **2013**, *64*, 249–256. [CrossRef] [PubMed]
7. Liao, C.H.; Kuo, H.C. Practical aspects of botulinum toxin-a treatment in patients with overactive bladder syndrome. *Int. Neurourol. J.* **2015**, *19*, 213–219. [CrossRef] [PubMed]
8. Liao, C.H.; Chen, S.F.; Kuo, H.C. Different number of intravesical onabotulinumtoxina injections for patients with refractory detrusor overactivity do not affect treatment outcome: A prospective randomized comparative study. *Neurourol. Urodyn.* **2016**, *35*, 717–723. [CrossRef]
9. Avallone, M.A.; Sack, B.S.; El-Arabi, A.; Guralnick, M.L.; O'Connor, R.C. Less is more-a pilot study evaluating one to three intradetrusor sites for injection of onabotulinumtoxina for neurogenic and idiopathic detrusor overactivity *Neurourol. Urodyn.* **2017**, *36*, 1104–1107. [CrossRef]
10. DiCarlo-Meacham, A.M.; Dengler, K.L.; Welch, E.K.; Brooks, D.I.; Gruber, D.D.; Osborn, D.J.; Scarlotta, L.; Vaccaro, C.M. Reduced versus standard intradetrusor onabotulinumtoxina injections for treatment of overactive bladder. *Neurourol. Urodyn.* **2023**, *42*, 366–374. [CrossRef]
11. Stewart, L.E.; Siddique, M.; Jacobs, K.M.; Raker, C.A.; Sung, V.W. Oral phenazopyridine vs intravesical lidocaine for bladder onabotulinumtoxina analgesia: A randomized controlled trial. *Am. J. Obstet. Gynecol.* **2022**, *227*, 308.e1–308.e8. [CrossRef]
12. Bickhaus, J.A.; Vaughan, M.; Truong, T.; Li, Y.J.; Siddiqui, N.Y. A comparison of antibiotic prophylaxis regimens to decrease the risk of post-procedure urinary tract infection after onabotulinum toxin a injection. *Int. Urogynecol. J.* **2020**, *31*, 1907–1912. [CrossRef] [PubMed]
13. White, N.; Iglesia, C.B. Overactive bladder. *Obstet. Gynecol. Clin. N. Am.* **2016**, *43*, 59–68. [CrossRef]
14. Kapur, A.; Harandi, A.A.; Cohen, T.; Ruan, H.; Dabrowski, C.; Anderson, R.; Hwang, K.; Lee, E.; Weissbart, S.; Kim, J. An analysis of factors that influence patient preference of third-line therapy for overactive bladder. *Neurourol. Urodyn.* **2022**, *41*, 1906–1913. [CrossRef]

15. Chapple, C.; Sievert, K.; MacDiarmid, S.; Khullar, V.; Radziszewski, P.; Nardo, C.; Thompson, C.; Zhou, J.; Haag-Molkenteller, C. Pivotal phase 3 study in overactive bladder (oab) patients with urinary incontinence confirms onabotulinumtoxina 100u significantly improves all oab symptoms and patients' quality of life. *Eur. Urol. Suppl.* **2013**, *1*, e741–e742. [CrossRef]
16. Kennelly, M.; Chapple, C.; Hale, D.; Sand, P.; Khullar, V. Expert consensus guidance on appropriate management of incomplete voiding of the bladder post-onabotulinumtoxina injection in patients with idiopathic overactive bladder. *EMJ Urol.* **2020**, *8*, 2–12.
17. Dmochowski, R.; Chapple, C.; Gruenenfelder, J.; Yu, J.; Patel, A.; Nelson, M.; Rovner, E. The effects of age, gender, and postvoid residual volume on catheterization rates after treatment with onabotulinumtoxina for overactive bladder. *Eur. Urol. Open Sci.* **2023**, *57*, 98–105. [CrossRef]
18. Cruz, F.; Herschorn, S.; Aliotta, P.; Brin, M.; Thompson, C.; Lam, W.; Daniell, G.; Heesakkers, J.; Haag-Molkenteller, C. Efficacy and safety of onabotulinumtoxina in patients with urinary incontinence due to neurogenic detrusor overactivity: A randomised, double-blind, placebo-controlled trial. *Eur. Urol.* **2011**, *60*, 742–750. [CrossRef] [PubMed]
19. Nitti, V.W.; Kohan, A.; McCammon, K.; Jenkins, B.; Ifantides, K.B.; Yushmanova, I.; Chapple, C. Efficacy and safety of onabotulinumtoxina for the treatment of overactive bladder in men and women: A pooled analysis. *Neurourol. Urodyn.* **2024**, *43*, 1765–1775. [CrossRef]
20. Bianchi, D.; Ricci, M.; Iacovelli, V.; Pletto, S.; Rosato, E.; Miano, R.; Agrò, E.F. Bladder onabotulinum toxin a injections and patients: Office-based vs. Operating room setting. *Continence* **2024**, *10*, 101227. [CrossRef]
21. Holmes, A.; O'Kane, D.; Wombwell, A.; Grills, R. Clinical utility of a single-use flexible cystoscope compared with a standard reusable device: A randomized noninferiority study. *J. Endourol.* **2023**, *37*, 80–84. [CrossRef]
22. Assmus, M.A.; Krambeck, A.E.; Lee, M.S.; Agarwal, D.K.; Mellon, M.; Rivera, M.E.; Large, T. Cost-effectiveness of 90-day single-use flexible cystoscope trial: Single center micro-costing analysis and user satisfaction. *Urology* **2022**, *167*, 61–66. [CrossRef] [PubMed]
23. Wen, X.; Shi, J.; Tan, W.; Jiang, H.; Wang, D.; Su, J.; Yang, G.; Zhang, B. Effects of aromatherapy and music therapy on patients' anxiety during MRI examinations: A randomized controlled trial. *Eur. Radiol.* **2023**, *33*, 2510–2518. [CrossRef]
24. Gange, S.N.; Baum, N. Verbal anesthesia: How and when to use it in urological procedures. *JOJ Urol. Nephrol.* **2018**, *4*, 555647.
25. Zargari Marandi, R.; Fjelsted, C.A.; Hrustanovic, I.; Dan Olesen, R.; Gazerani, P. Eye movements in response to pain-related feelings in the presence of low and high cognitive loads. *Behav. Sci.* **2020**, *10*, 92. [CrossRef] [PubMed]
26. Lightner, D.J.; Wymer, K.; Sanchez, J.; Kavoussi, L. Best practice statement on urologic procedures and antimicrobial prophylaxis *J. Urol.* **2020**, *203*, 351–356. [CrossRef]
27. Eckhardt, S.E.; Takashima, Y.; Handler, S.J.; Tenggardjaja, C.; Yazdany, T. Antibiotic regimen and route of administration do not alter rates of urinary tract infection after intravesical botulinum toxin injection for overactive bladder. *Int. Urogynecol. J.* **2022**, *33* 703–709. [CrossRef]
28. Mensah, E.E.; Toia, B.; Nguyen, L.; Hamid, R.; Pakzad, M.; Ockrim, J.L.; Walker, R.; Greenwell, T.J.; Nitkunan, T.; Sharma, D.; et al Intravesical onabotulinumtoxina injections in patients on antiplatelet and anticoagulation therapy. *Neurourol. Urodyn.* **2021**, *40* 1829–1833. [CrossRef]
29. Shenot, P.J.; Mark, J.R. Intradetrusor onabotulinumtoxina injection: How I do it. *Can. J. Urol.* **2013**, *20*, 6649–6655.
30. MacDiarmid, S.; Glazier, D.B.; McCrery, R.J.; Kennelly, M.J.; Nelson, M.; Ifantides, K.B.; McCammon, K.A. Efficacy and safety of an alternative onabotulinumtoxina injection paradigm for refractory overactive bladder. *Neurourol. Urodyn.* **2024**, *43*, 31–43 [CrossRef]
31. Bernstein, S.; Schwartz, M.; Ifantides, K.B. Patient persistence to onabotulinumtoxina treatment for overactive bladder using a reduced-injection-site paradigm: A retrospective chart review study. *Toxicon* **2024**, *237*, 107368. [CrossRef]
32. Ton, J.; Downing, P.; Versi, E.; van Uem, S.; Ephraim, S.; Murphy, M.; Lucente, V. Outcomes of a single trigone-only vs. 20 trigone-sparing injections of onabotulinumtoxina for refractory overactive bladder (oab). *Int. Urol. Nephrol.* **2021**, *53*, 1067–1072 [CrossRef] [PubMed]
33. Cui, Y.; Cai, T.; Dong, T.; Zhang, X.; Zhou, Z.; Lu, Y.; Zhang, Y.; Wu, J.; Gao, Z.; Wang, Y.; et al. Trigonal-sparing vs. Trigonal-involved onabotulinumtoxina injection for the treatment of overactive bladder: A systematic review and meta-analysis. *Front. Neurol.* **2021**, *12*, 651635. [CrossRef]
34. Purves, J.T.; Spruill, L.; Rovner, E.; Borisko, E.; McCants, A.; Mugo, E.; Wingard, A.; Trusk, T.C.; Bacro, T.; Hughes, F.M., Jr. A three dimensional nerve map of human bladder trigone. *Neurourol. Urodyn.* **2017**, *36*, 1015–1019. [CrossRef] [PubMed]
35. Ramirez-Castaneda, J.; Jankovic, J. Long-term efficacy, safety, and side effect profile of botulinum toxin in dystonia: A 20-year follow-up. *Toxicon* **2014**, *90*, 344–348. [CrossRef]
36. Osman, N.I.; Chapple, C.R. Overactive bladder syndrome: Current pathophysiological concepts and therapeutic approaches *Arab. J. Urol.* **2013**, *11*, 313–318. [CrossRef] [PubMed]
37. Chapple, C.; Patel, A. Botulinum toxin--new mechanisms, new therapeutic directions? *Eur. Urol.* **2006**, *49*, 606–608. [CrossRef]

38. Szczypior, M.; Połom, W.; Wąż, P.; Matuszewski, M. Application of methylene blue as an improvement of the injection technique of botulinum toxin a in the treatment of refractory idiopathic overactive bladder: Prospective, single-blind (patient-blind), randomized trial. *Wideochir Inne Tech Maloinwazyjne* **2019**, *14*, 420–426. [CrossRef]
39. Freemantle, N.; Ginsberg, D.A.; McCool, R.; Fleetwood, K.; Arber, M.; Khalaf, K.; Loveman, C.; Ni, Q.; Glanville, J. Comparative assessment of onabotulinumtoxina and mirabegron for overactive bladder: An indirect treatment comparison. *BMJ Open* **2016**, *6*, e009122. [CrossRef]
40. McCammon, K.; Gousse, A.; Kohan, A.; Glazier, D.; Gruenenfelder, J.; Bai, Z.; Patel, A.; Hale, D. Early and consistent improvements in urinary symptoms and quality of life with onabotulinumtoxina in patients with overactive bladder and urinary incontinence: Results from a randomized, placebo-controlled, phase iv clinical trial. *Female Pelvic Med. Reconstr. Surg.* **2021**, *27*, 450–456. [CrossRef]
41. Cox, L.; Cameron, A.P. Onabotulinumtoxina for the treatment of overactive bladder. *Res. Rep. Urol.* **2014**, *6*, 79–89. [CrossRef]

toxins

MDPI

Review

Intravesical Onabotulinum Toxin A Injection Paradigms for Idiopathic Overactive Bladder: A Scoping Review of Clinical Outcomes, Techniques, and Implications for Practice and Future Research

Ekene Enemchukwu [1,*], Hodan Mohamud [2], Shada Sinclair [1], Victoria Harbour [1], Raveen Syan [3], Michael Kennelly and Susanna Gunamany [1]

1 Department of Urology, Stanford School of Medicine, Palo Alto, CA 94304, USA; sssinc@stanford.edu (S.S.); vharbour@stanford.edu (V.H.); susannag@stanford.edu (S.G.)
2 Temerty Faculty of Medicine, University of Toronto, Toronto, ON M5S1A1, Canada; hodan.mohamud@mail.utoronto.ca
3 Department of Urology, Miller School of Medicine, University of Miami, Miami, FL 33136, USA; raveen.syan@med.miami.edu
4 Department of Urology, Atrium Health—Carolinas Medical Center, Wake Forest University School of Medicine, Winston-Salem, NC 27101, USA; michael.kennelly@atriumhealth.org
* Correspondence: enemche@stanford.edu

Abstract

Introduction and Objectives: Onabotulinum toxin A (BTXA) is an effective treatment for refractory idiopathic overactive bladder (iOAB). Given the wide spectrum of patient factors and combination of symptoms, a tailored approach to management is needed. This scoping review assesses injection paradigms for iOAB. Prior studies have established the safety and efficacy of BTXA injections, and this review focuses on exploring variations in injection techniques that may inform more tailored approaches and support future research toward optimizing patient outcomes. Methods: We conducted a systematic literature search. Inclusion criteria included full-text English language and primary research studies assessing outcomes in adults undergoing BTXA for iOAB. Findings are summarized using narrative synthesis. Results: Forty-three articles were identified. Key findings include fewer injections (1–10 vs. 20–40) maintains efficacy while reducing procedure time, discomfort, and retreatment hesitancy. Durability appears to be lower with suburothelial and bladder base injections and higher with detrusor and bladder body injections, though these may carry an increased risk of urinary retention requiring clean intermittent catheterization. Trigone inclusion appears safe and effective without increased vesicoureteral reflux risk. Conclusions: Study heterogeneity and inconsistent reporting limit strong conclusions. Included injection paradigms demonstrated efficacy, high tolerability, symptom relief, and quality-of-life improvements with few adverse events. Further research is needed to refine optimal injection strategies to enhance patient comfort, maximize efficacy, and minimize adverse events. Future studies should ensure comprehensive data collection to clarify these associations.

Keywords: onabotulinumtoxinA intravesical injection; urge urinary incontinence; overactive bladder; idiopathic; injection paradigm; trigone; suburothelial

Key Contribution: This study highlights an opportunity to leverage our knowledge of BTXA's mechanism of action to optimize outcomes, with an emphasis on the need for further exploration of the impact of injection number, site, and depth. Additionally, it calls for investigating how these factors impact specific patient populations, considering factors such as age, gender, comorbidities, urodynamic parameters, and prior BTXA therapy. Based on our findings, we recommend that future research focus on tailoring injection doses, number, and sites to specific iOAB subgroups to balance treatment efficacy, adverse events, and tolerability, potentially reducing patient hesitancy. We also propose the development of a minimum data set to guide and standardize future investigations and reporting.

1. Introduction

Overactive bladder (OAB) is a chronic, debilitating condition characterized by urinary urgency, frequency, and nocturia with or without urgency urinary incontinence (UUI) occurring in the absence of other pathology [1]. The reported prevalence of OAB varies widely, between 16.5% and 43% in the United States [2–5], and increases with age [4,6,7]. It negatively impacts health-related quality of life (QOL), productivity, sleep, sexual health, and mental well-being [8,9].

Evidence-based guideline-recommended treatments, include behavioral therapy, pelvic floor exercises, pharmacotherapy, and minimally invasive therapies. The recent 2024 American Urological Association (AUA) and Society of Urodynamics, Female Pelvic Medicine and Urogenital Reconstruction (SUFU) OAB guidelines emphasize shared decision-making to incorporate patient goals and identify the most appropriate therapy or combination of therapies for each patient [10]. This encourages a more tailored approach to OAB management by considering the patient's specific symptoms, needs, values, and preferences. This paradigm shift highlights the need for rigorous study of tailored OAB therapies to optimize outcomes and minimize adverse effects.

1.1. BTXA Mechanism of Action

Our understanding of onabotulinum toxin A's (BTXA) mechanism of action offers a unique opportunity to tailor therapy based on idiopathic OAB (iOAB) phenotype and other individual patient factors. BTXA acts on synaptic vesicle glycoprotein (SV2), present on over 90% of parasympathetic nerve fibers in the detrusor muscle and approximately half of the sensory nerve fibers in the suburothelium [11,12]. When BTXA binds SV2 at the neuromuscular junction, it inhibits the release of acetylcholine and reduces ATP and substance P release, reducing bladder contractility and the micturition reflex [8,11,12].

The normal bladder wall is 3–6 mm thick and consists of the urothelium, suburothelium, detrusor muscle, and adventitia, each supporting its function [13]. The layers of the bladder play a key role in function by integrating sensory and motor signaling. Presynaptic nerve terminals for sensory function are primarily in the suburothelium, which contains a dense network of afferent fibers mediating bladder filling and urgency. Motor function is controlled by parasympathetic efferent nerves in the detrusor muscle, where acetylcholine release activates muscarinic receptors to facilitate detrusor contraction. Understanding the precise location of these presynaptic nerve fibers is key to optimizing BTXA placement, allowing us to target sensory and motor components of bladder function. Once BTXA is internalized by a presynaptic nerve, it can only affect that specific nerve, concentrating its effects within that nerve. However, if BTXA spreads across multiple nerve terminals, therapeutic outcomes are expected to be more significant.

While trigone-sparing techniques were initially employed to minimize extravesical spread and the theoretical risk of vesicoureteral reflux (VUR), studies have not shown an increased risk of VUR with trigonal injections [14,15]. This is particularly relevant given the unique anatomy of the trigone. Unlike the bladder walls, the trigone lacks detrusor muscle fibers, but it contains a dense network of sensory fibers expressing SV2 that contribute to the sensory arm of the micturition reflex. Targeting these sensory nerves in the trigone may enhance efficacy while reducing the risk of urinary retention in high-risk iOAB populations [16]. Additionally, the number, volume, and location of injections may impact pain, tolerability, and therapy adherence rates [17].

1.2. Rationale for Injection Paradigms

BTXA is an effective, Food and Drug Administration (FDA)-approved therapy for the management of idiopathic OAB (iOAB) that has demonstrated clinical efficacy and safety in two pivotal phase III trials that utilized an intradetrusor, low-volume (0.5 mL), 20-injection, trigone-sparing injection paradigm [8,11]. This injection technique has been shown to significantly reduce urinary urgency and UUI episodes, with meaningful improvements in QOL and a low risk of transient urinary retention, hematuria, and urinary tract infection (UTI).

Many injection paradigms have been described, varying in injection depth (suburothelium vs. detrusor), site (trigone vs. trigone-sparing vs. bladder base vs. detrusor), number, volume, BTXA concentration, and needle size. Currently, there is no consensus on the optimal injection paradigm, and previous reviews have been limited by the exclusion of males and the inclusion of mixed populations with idiopathic overactive bladder (iOAB) and neurogenic detrusor overactivity (NDO) [18–20]. This scoping review provides an overview of the current literature on the efficacy of various intravesical BTXA injection paradigms for adults with iOAB, focusing on clinical outcomes and adverse events. It aims to clarify the impact of different injection parameters, identify research gaps, and propose suggestions for future investigation.

2. Results

Of 1991 records, 43 studies met the inclusion criteria (Table 1) and were included (Figure 1), representing 6740 study participants, avoiding duplication from secondary analyses. Of these, 82.4% were women, with a mean age of 62.7. Supplemental Table S1 provides an overview of the injection paradigm characteristics and outcomes. Supplemental Table S2 details the following parameters: site and depth of injection, number of injections, and volume/concentration.

Table 1. Inclusion and Exclusion Criteria.

Inclusion Criteria	Exclusion Criteria
Human Subjects, Adults (>18 years), Male and Female	Non-English language
Idiopathic Overactive Bladder	Neurogenic bladder
OnabotulinumtoxinA	Other types of botulinum toxins
Primary research articles	Case studies, Systematic reviews, Meta-analysis, Scoping reviews, Abstracts, Conference Abstracts, Case studies and Editorials
Outcomes: Efficacy, Adverse Events	Full text is not available or retrievable

Injection Protocols: The majority of included studies used a 100–200 U dose (range: 50 U–300 U) of BTXA, administered in 0.5 mL (range: 0.2–10 mL) aliquots across 20 injection sites (range: 1–40) into the detrusor wall, sparing the trigone, under local anesthesia with a rigid or flexible cystoscope and a 23-gauge needle (Supplemental Tables S1 and S2).

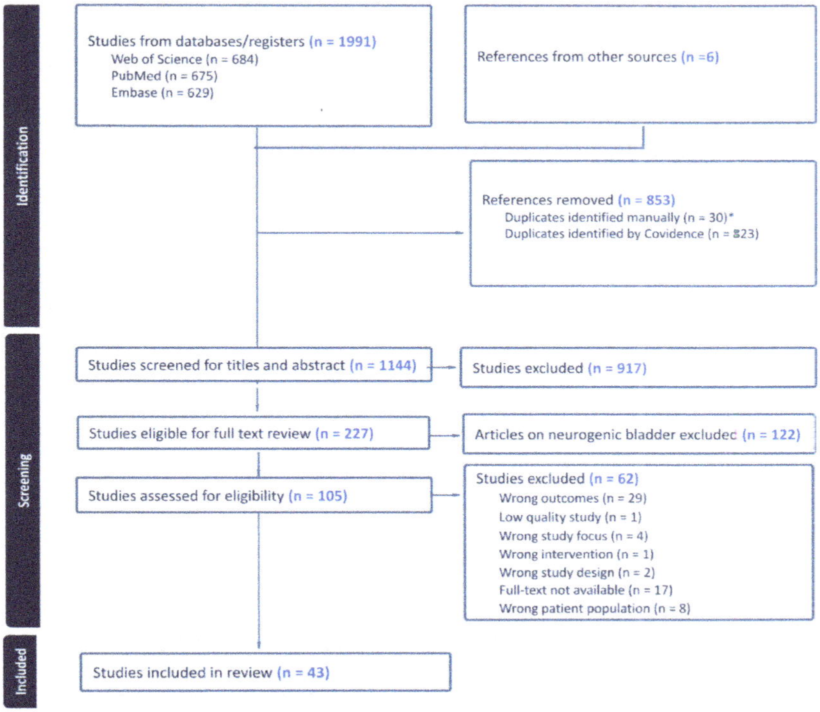

Figure 1. PRISMA flow diagram depicting the study selection process. * Jiang et al. (2017) [21] were excluded as duplicates due to the identical patient population, treatment, outcomes, and findings of Hsiao et al. (2016) [22].

2.1. Dose Efficacy and Adverse Events

The current FDA-approved starting dose for intravesical BTXA is 100 U, which can be increased to 200 U with inadequate response [23]. This recommendation is based on a phase II randomized trial by Dmochowski et al. (2010), which identified a dose–response relationship in UUI rates with minimal improvement beyond 150 U and reduced efficacy at 50 U. Most studies (35 of 43, or 81.4%) included in this review assessed the 100 U dose of BTX alone or as a treatment arm [8,9,11,14,22,24–54]. Three studies assessed the impact of 50 U (3/43; 6.9%) [9,24,52], six assessed 150 U (6/43: 14%) [9,24,26,38,51,52], fourteen assessed 200 U (14/43: 32.5%) [9,15,24,25,29,39,40,44,45,52,55–58], and six included doses exceeding 200 U (4/43; 9.3%) [9,24,29,38,52,56] (Supplemental Table S1).

50 U Dose: In a phase II placebo-controlled, randomized, dose-ranging trial (n = 313) [24,52], changes in UUI episodes/week and urodynamic parameters were assessed in placebo, 50 U, 100 U, 150 U, 200 U, and 300 U groups. The 50 U dose outperformed the placebo in UUI resolution (15.9% vs. 29.8%), but demonstrated both reduced and less sustained efficacy outcomes compared to the 100 U or higher doses (37–57%). However, the 50 U dose exhibited the lowest rates of adverse events, including urinary retention with the need for clean intermittent catheterization (CIC) (5.4% vs. 10.9–12.2%). (Supplemental Table S1) Patient-reported outcomes highlight this limited efficacy [9], with no significant benefit in health-related QOL improvements when compared to placebo, while higher doses (>100 U) demonstrated significant improvements [9]. Overall, the 50 U dose reduced adverse events, but provided poorly sustained, limited urodynamic efficacy and HRQOL improvements.

100 U Dose: The dose–response relationship observed in the phase II trials identified 100 U as the optimal balance of symptom improvement and adverse events [9,24,52]. The 100 U dose offered superior efficacy in UUI resolution compared to 50 U (50 U: 29.8% vs. 100 U: 37%), with minimal additional benefit observed at the 150 U dose (40.8%). Similarly, adverse events, such as elevated PVR requiring CIC, were dose-dependent, but less frequent at 100 U (10.9%) compared to higher doses (150 U: 20%, 200 U: 21.2%, 300 U: 16.4%) [52]. Phase III and IV trials confirmed the safety and efficacy of 100 U, with high UUI resolution rates (28.9–32%) and low CIC rates (6.1–6.9%) [8,11,12].

150 U Dose: In a small RCT (n = 42), Cohen et al. (2009) observed no differences between 100 U and 150 U doses in clinical outcomes, including dry rates, urodynamic parameters, QOL, urinary retention requiring CIC (n = 2, 1 in each group), or UTI [38]. Similarly, in a 3.5-year extension of the phase II and III BTXA trials, Nitti et al. (2016) (n = 829) observed equivalent outcomes in the 286 patients who received 150 U and the remainder of the cohort who received 100 U [26]. These studies support prior findings that 150 U offers no additional benefit over 100 U, demonstrating similar improvements in OAB symptoms, urodynamic parameters, and QOL, but with a higher risk of CIC.

200 U Dose: In an RCT, Amundsen et al. (2016) compared BTX-A, 200 U, and sacral neuromodulation (SNM) for refractory UUI in women [57]. At 6 months, BTX-A showed a significant reduction in UUI episodes (−3.9 vs. −3.25, $p < 0.01$) and higher UUI resolution rates (20% vs. 4%, $p < 0.001$) vs. SNM. Both groups reported similar patient-perceived improvement (71% vs. 68%, $p = 0.82$). Adverse events were more frequent with BTX-A, including UTI (35% vs. 11%, $p < 0.001$) and elevated PVR requiring CIC (2.1% vs. 0%, $p = 0.04$). Other studies also demonstrated significant reductions in UUI at the 200 U dose vs. placebo (−57.5 vs. 9.3%) ($p < 0.01$) [56], with low (4.5%) CIC rates. CIC rates (18–21.2%) vary across studies, often depending on how urinary retention requiring CIC was defined [39,52].

Special Populations: Older Adults: BTXA 100 U is effective in older adults. In a retrospective study (n = 192), Ou et al. (2023) reported similar subjective cure rates: 66.9% in younger (<75 years) and 60% in older (≥75 years) patients with iOAB. Adverse event rates, including urinary retention (8.7% vs. 12.3%, $p = 0.42$) and UTI (14.2% vs. 9.2%, $p = 0.33$), were comparable between groups [41].

Summary: The 100 U dose of BTXA is optimal, with minimal additional improvement at 150 U and reduced efficacy at 50 U. Higher doses, such as 200 U, offer higher symptom relief, but carry a higher risk of CIC, while 100 U appears to be equally effective in both "younger" and "older" adults. Further studies are needed to determine which iOAB population may benefit from the alternative doses (e.g., 50 U dose) to reduce AE risk.

2.2. Site and Depth of Injection

2.2.1. Outcomes Based on the Depth of Injection (Suburothelial vs. Detrusor)

There is a paucity of studies evaluating the impact of injection depth on treatment outcomes, with only two studies meeting the inclusion criteria for this review. In an RCT of refractory iOAB (n = 45), Kuo (2007) compared three injection techniques using 100 U BTXA: trigone-sparing detrusor, trigone-sparing suburothelial, and trigone-including bladder base suburothelial injections [14] (Figure 2). At 3 months, there were no statistically significant differences in efficacy ($p = 0.07$) or QOL improvement ($p = 0.56$) between groups (Figure 3). However, detrusor injections were more durable than suburothelial bladder body injections, followed by suburothelial bladder base injections (Figure 3). Urinary retention requiring CIC occurred more frequently in the detrusor (n = 2, 13.3%) and suburothelial bladder body (n = 2, 13.3%) groups than the suburothelial bladder base group (0%). No VUR was observed. In a subsequent study (n = 105), Kuo (2011) compared trigone-sparing detrusor, bladder body/trigone, and bladder base/trigone injections, finding no significant difference in success rates at 3, 6, or 9 months. At 12 months, the bladder base/trigone group had numerically lower success rates (37%) than the bladder body (49%) and bladder body/trigone (50%) groups, though these differences were not statistically significant. CIC rates were 0% for bladder base, 5% for bladder body, and 11% for bladder body/trigone, though the study was underpowered [53].

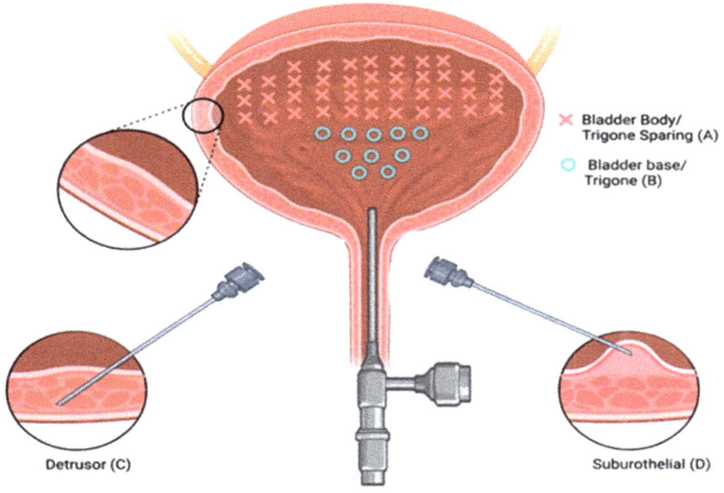

Figure 2. Three types of intravesical botulinum toxin A injections. Intravesical injections at 40 sites with trigone sparing (A) using suburothelial injection (D) and/or detrusor injection (C). Bladder base and trigonal injections (B) were performed at 10 sites.

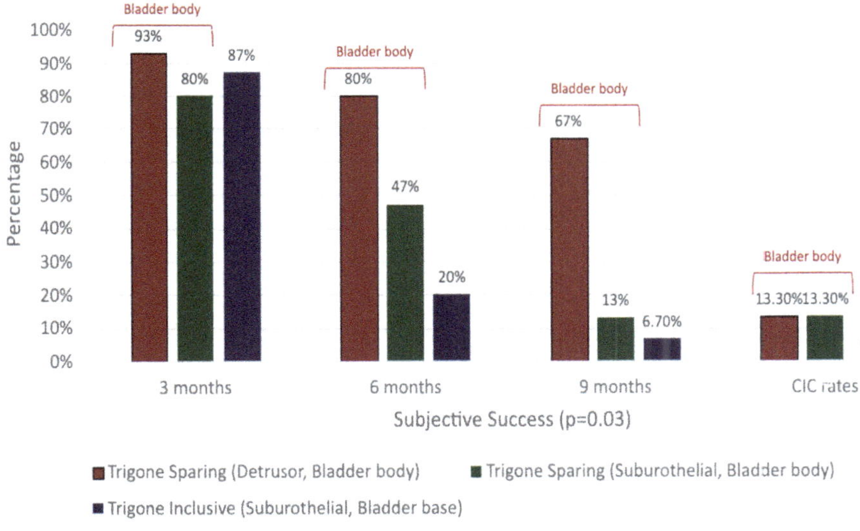

Figure 3. Comparison of clinical outcomes in detrusor, suburothelial, and bladder base injections.

Overall, BTXA demonstrates efficacy independently of the injection depth [31,33,51]. Suburothelial and bladder base injections may be less durable but have lower CIC rates than detrusor or bladder body injections. Bladder base/trigone injections may also be less durable than bladder body injections, regardless of trigone involvement, but with the benefit of lower CIC rates.

Summary: Detrusor injections are likely more durable than suburothelial injections, though they were associated with higher rates of urinary retention requiring CIC. In contrast, suburothelial injections improved symptoms with a lower risk of CIC.

2.2.2. Trigone-Sparing vs. Trigone-Including Injection Paradigms

Most studies in this review focused on the impact of trigone-sparing injection techniques, with only eight (8/43; 18.6%) examining trigone-including injections in patients with iOAB [14,15,32,35,37,48,53,57].

2.2.3. Trigone-Sparing Detrusor Injections vs. Trigone-Including Detrusor Injections

El-Hefnawy et al. (2021) conducted an RCT (n = 103) comparing trigone-sparing (n = 52) and trigone-including (n = 51) injections, administering 100 U BTXA in 20 (0.5 mL) sites via a 7-gauge needle [37]. Both groups demonstrated significant reductions in OABSS scores, with UI episodes reduced by 93% in the trigone-sparing group and 85% in the trigone-inclusive group (p = 0.38). Adverse events were more common in the trigone-inclusive group, with 19.6% reporting voiding difficulties and 3.9% requiring CIC for PVR >200 mL, but there were no differences in UTI rates or VUR between groups [37].

In a retrospective cohort study (n = 45), Ton et al. compared 100 U BTXA administered as a single 10 mL trigone-only injection (n = 19) vs. 20 trigone-sparing 0.5 mL injections (n = 26) [48]. Both groups had similar durability and adverse event rates, but the trigone-only group had a lower PVR (113 mL vs. 160 mL, $p < 0.02$), a lower CIC rate (5.3% vs. 17.4%, $p < 0.02$), and shorter procedure times (4.3 min vs. 5.7 min, $p < 0.01$). No VUR was observed. In an RCT, Kuo (2007) (see Section 2.2.1) observed superior durability in outcomes in the trigone-sparing bladder body (detrusor and suburothelial) group compared to the trigone-inclusive bladder base group (p = 0.01, Figure 3, Supplemental Table S2). However, CIC rates were lower in the trigone-inclusive group (0% vs. 13.3%), with no VUR observed [14].

2.2.4. Trigone-Inclusive Detrusor Injections vs. Placebo

MacDiarmid et al. (2023) explored an alternative injection paradigm using ten injections (1.0 mL), eight administered to the posterior wall and two to the bladder trigone [35]. In this phase IV multicenter, randomized, double-blind, placebo-controlled trial (n = 120), the BTXA group demonstrated significantly greater reductions in daily UI episodes at week 12 (−2.9) vs. placebo (−0.3) ($p < 0.0001$). Trigonal injections were generally well tolerated, with low adverse events rates in both groups (UTI: 15.4% vs. 5.1%, CIC: 2.6% vs. 0%, dysuria: 5.1% vs. 2.6%, in BTXA vs. placebo, respectively). VUR was not reported [35].

2.2.5. Trigone-Inclusive Injections vs. No Comparator

Onem et al. (2018) conducted a multicenter, prospective single-arm study (n = 80) to investigate the efficacy and safety of administering 100 U BTXA in 20 injections (0.5 mL), including the trigone [32]. At 3 months, bladder diary parameters (UUI, urgency, and urinary frequency) and urinary incontinence QOL (I-QOL) scores showed significant improvements from baseline ($p < 0.05$). The treatment satisfaction rate was 82.5%. Adverse events included uncomplicated UTI (6.25%) and hematuria (6.25%), and CIC was initiated in three patients (3.8%). VUR was not reported.

Summary: Trigone-inclusive protocols demonstrate good efficacy, no VUR, and low adverse event rates. One study suggests that patients are more likely to experience subjective voiding difficulties with trigone inclusion, while two others indicate that retention rates are lower when the trigone is included. However, the heterogeneity in trigone injection techniques across studies (e.g., trigone only, trigone with bladder base, or trigone with detrusor) limits the ability to draw meaningful differences in adverse events.

2.3. *Number of Injections*

Studies have explored pain reduction strategies for the administration of BTXA, including minimizing injection sites [17]. Thirty-eight studies (90.5%) reported the number of BTXA injections administered. Most (n = 22/43; 51.2%) used a standard 20-injection technique [8,9,11,14,22,25–32,34,36–38,42,45,52,56,57], which consistently improved outcomes (frequency, nocturia, urgency, dry rates, and QOL) compared to baseline or placebo [8,9,22,25–32,34,36–38,42,45,52,53,56,57]. Seven studies reported significant improvements in QOL [8,9,12,26,27,32,40]. Alternative injection regimens (e.g., 10, 30, 40 injections) were also evaluated, with some directly comparing injection paradigms (e.g., 5 vs. 20 injection sites) [42,43,47]. Pain scores were assessed in only three studies [42,47,49].

2.3.1. 10 vs. 40 Injections

In an RCT (n = 45), Kuo (2007) (see Section 2.2.1) compared 100 U BTXA administered via 40 detrusor, 40 suburothelial, and 10 suburothelial bladder base injections [14]. The 40-injection groups had more durable success rates, but also experienced higher CIC rates compared to the 10-injection group (n = 4/30; 13.3% vs. 0%). However, since injection sites varied across groups, the relative impact of injection number vs. location remains unclear. Pain scores and procedure duration were not assessed.

2.3.2. 10 vs. 20 vs. 40 Injections

In an RCT, Liao et al. (2016) compared 10, 20, and 40 suburothelial BTXA injections (100 U dose) [43]. The 10- and 40-injection groups demonstrated significant reductions in UUI episodes at 6 months, with decreases of 7.24 episodes/day (8.95 $\pm$ 10.74 to 1.71 $\pm$ 2.34) and 4.53 episodes/day (9.86 $\pm$ 13.11 to 5.33 $\pm$ 12.17), respectively, while the 20-injection group showed no significant change (decrease of 0.15 from 5.29 $\pm$ 7.64 to 5.44 $\pm$ 16.66). UTI rates were higher in the 20-injection group (31.8%) compared to the 10 (12.5%) and 40-injection groups (9.5%), with no significant differences in other adverse events. Pain scores or duration of procedures were not assessed.

2.3.3. 5 vs. 20 Injection Sites (2 Studies)

DiCarlo-Meacham et al. (2023) conducted a randomized noninferiority trial (n = 77) comparing 100 U BTXA given in 5 "reduced" injections (2 mL/site) vs. 20 "standard" injections (0.5 mL/site) [42]. There was a significant improvement in both arms on validated questionnaires (p < 0.001) and overall treatment success of 68% with no statistically significant difference between groups. Urinary retention requiring CIC was observed in the 5-injection group (n = 2, 4.9%), but not in the 20-injection group. There was no difference in UTI rates (p = 0.28). Both groups had similar pain scores, but the "reduced" 5-injection group was more willing to repeat the procedure (odds ratio = 3.8, 95% CI: 1.42–10.67, p = 0.004).

Chang et al. conducted an RCT (n = 60) comparing pain and procedure time in patients with iOAB receiving 100 units of BTXA in 5 injections vs. 20 injections [47]. Patients rated their pain on a 10-point visual analogue scale (VAS), and procedure time was recorded. Results showed no significant difference in pain scores between the groups (p = 0.27), but the 5-injection group had a significantly shorter procedure time (76 s vs. 176 s, p < 0 001). There were no differences in subjective efficacy between the 5- and 20-injection groups (+2 vs. +2 on the Global Response Assessment (GRA) score) or adverse events between groups

(UTI: 20% vs. 16.7% and CIC: 10% vs. 6.7%), respectively [47]. VAS scores were also similar between treatment-naïve and repeat-treatment patients ($p = 0.27$).

2.3.4. 10 vs. 20 Injection Sites

In a single-blinded randomized trial, Zdroik et al. evaluated the effect of BTXA injection number and volume (100 U delivered as ten 1 mL injections vs. twenty 0.5 mL injections) on procedural pain using an 11-point numerical pain rating scale (NPRS) immediately after the procedure [49]. Local anesthesia was administered pre-procedurally via bupivacaine and $NaHCO_3$ bladder instillation. The median pain scores were reported as 4 (interquartile range: 1.5–5) for the 10-injection group and 3 (interquartile range: 1–4) for the 20-injection group, with no statistically significant difference observed between the two groups ($p = 0.82$) [49]. There were no significant differences in efficacy (success rates: 46.7% vs. 40%, $p = 0.8$) or safety (UTI: 2/19 (10.5%) vs. 2/21 (9.5%), CIC: 1/21 (4.8%) vs. 2/19 (10.5%) in the 10- and 20-injection group, respectively).

2.3.5. 1 Injections vs. 20 Injections

In a retrospective cohort study, Ton et al. (see Section 2.2.3) assessed differences in outcomes for BTXA 100 U given in a single trigonal injection vs. 20 trigone-sparing injections [48]. The authors observed no significant differences in inter-injection intervals or UTI rates between groups. However, the single-injection (trigone only) group had lower rates of urinary retention requiring catheterization (5.3% vs. 17.4%, ($p = 0.014$)). Procedure time was lower in the single-injection group (4.3 ± 2.02, 5.7 ± 2.9, $p = 0.003$). Differences in pain scores were not assessed or reported [48].

2.3.6. 30 Injections

In a prospective cohort study, Okamura et al. (2013) evaluated ($n = 17$) participants with idiopathic OAB who were treated with 100 U BTXA reconstituted in 15 mL of 0.9% normal saline and injected 0.5 mL for a total of 30 submucosal injections. They observed a significant reduction in urinary frequency, urgency, and urgency urinary incontinence, with no adverse events reported [33]. No episodes of urinary retention or catheterization were observed. Pain was not assessed.

Summary: While injection number alone does not appear to impact efficacy, it is important to consider BTXA's mechanism of action, as other factors such as volume, distribution, depth, and location all contribute to efficacy. Given that injection volume and number are interconnected, caution is warranted in attributing efficacy solely to the number of injections. One study found that five injections were associated with a greater willingness to repeat the procedure, even though pain scores were similar for higher numbers of injections.

2.4. Dilution and Volume

2.4.1. Dilution

Among the 43 studies, 34 (79%) reported data on the volume and dilution of BTXA injections, of which 13 administered 0.5 mL per injection with 10 U/mL concentrations. Studies employing this volume and concentration demonstrated significant improvements in OAB symptoms, including reductions in urgency, micturition episodes, nocturia, and improved QOL scores compared to baseline or placebo groups [8,11,12,14,25–27,37,41–44,52]. Adverse events commonly reported in these studies included UTIs, dysuria, bacteriuria, urinary retention, hematuria, and the need for CIC.

One study with an alternative BTXA dilution strategy met the inclusion criteria for this review (see Section 2.3.6). In a prospective cohort study with no comparison group, Okamura et al. (2013) evaluated ($n = 17$) participants treated with 100 U BTXA reconstituted in 15 mL (6.6 U/mL) and injected 0.5 mL (3.3 U/injection) for a total of 30 submucosal injections. They observed a significant reduction in urinary frequency, urgency, and urgency urinary incontinence, with no urinary retention reported [33].

2.4.2. Volume

2.4.2.1. mL vs. 2 mL Injection Volume

Chang et al. (see Section 2.3.3) compared the 100 U BTXA dose ($n = 40$) administered as either 2 mL (5 injections) or 0.5 mL (20 injections) aliquots. Pain scores were similar between groups ($p = 0.27$), but procedure time was significantly shorter with higher volume injections (fewer injections) (76 s vs. 176 s; $p < 0.001$). No differences in GRA score (efficacy) or adverse events were observed [47].

2.4.2.2. mL vs. 1 mL Injection Volume

In a single-blinded randomized trial, Zdroik et al. (see Section 2.3.4) compared the outcomes of 100 units of BTXA administered in 1 mL (10 injections) vs. 0.5 mL (20 injections) aliquots. There was no difference in efficacy ($p = 0.82$), adverse events, or NPRS scores immediately after the procedure ($p = 0.84$) [49].

2.4.2.3. mL vs. 10 mL Injection Volume

In a single-institution, retrospective chart review, Ton et al. (see Section 2.2.3) compared outcomes for 100 U BTXA administered in a single 10 mL injection into the trigone vs. 0.5 mL (20 injections) in a trigone-sparing injection pattern. However, in the trigone-only group, the needle was tunneled intramurally towards the dome, and methylene blue was used for visualization and observation of spread in both groups, though the degree of spread was not measured. The procedure setting or method of anesthesia was not reported. While there were no differences in GRA scores, the high-volume (10 mL), single-injection group had significantly shorter procedure time (4.3 min vs. 5.7 min, $p < 0.01$). However, anesthetic details and pain scores were not reported. In addition, the differences observed in PVR outcomes were not clinically significant (113 ± 111(0–500) vs. 160 ± 134(0–850); however, it is unclear if these observed differences were the result of the location (trigone) or localization (volume/number) of the injection [48].

Summary: There are no head-to-head studies comparing different injection volumes with the same dose and number of injections, but BTXA has proven effective at various volumes and concentrations. While using higher volumes with fewer injections reduces procedure time, the 1.4 min difference may not be clinically significant and should be weighed against patient tolerability, which was not formally assessed or reported.

2.5. Needle Size

Needle size has traditionally been discussed in the context of safety. In more contemporary literature, needle size has been explored as a potential contributor to pain and tolerability of BTXA therapy under local anesthesia [17].

There is limited literature available assessing the impact of injection needle size on intradetrusor BTXA outcomes and adverse events. Current recommendations are for an ultrafine needle (22 to 27 gauge and 4 mm long) to mitigate the risk of bladder wall perforation or inadvertent extravesical administration of BTXA [19,59,60]. The normal bladder wall is 4–6 mm, and consequently most commercially available needles are 2–5 mm in length. Retractable needles are available to help compress and tamponade any areas of significant bleeding.

However, few studies report needle size or length, and none of the studies included in this review directly compared needle sizes, with only 8 out of 42 studies (19%) specifying the injection needle used [14,28,36–38,43,45,56]. Various sizes were reported, including

7 gauge by El Hefnawy et al., performed under sedation (n = 1) [37]. Other sizes included 18-gauge (n = 1), 22-gauge (n = 2), 23-gauge (n = 3), and 27-gauge (n = 1) needles. Despite the variance in needle size, all eight studies reported a significant improvement in clinical and QOL endpoints compared to baseline or placebo groups. Notably, there were no discernible differences in adverse events, such as hematuria or UTI, relative to injection needle size. Pain scores were not routinely reported in these studies.

Summary: Needles come in several sizes and lengths, flexible vs. rigid and retractable vs. fixed. Overall, needle size does not appear to directly impact efficacy or safety, though the studies available are too few in number to draw any meaningful conclusions on the impact of needle size on efficacy outcomes.

2.6. Scope Type

In the literature, flexible cystoscopy is reported to be more comfortable and generally preferred [61,62] compared to rigid cystoscopy for both men [63,64] and women [65] of all age groups. Other studies report negligible differences in pain perception between the two methods, suggesting that differences in tolerance may be minimal [66–68]. However, rigid scopes are generally easier to use, have a lower learning curve, and offer better control, improved visualization, and greater precision. They are also typically less expensive and have lower maintenance costs. All studies included in this review used rigid, flexible, or a combination of both cystoscope types. Recorded cystoscope sizes ranged from 14 to 23 French. None of the included studies investigated the effect of scope type (rigid vs. flexible) or size on ease of therapy administration, therapy outcomes, or patient tolerability (e.g., pain scores). However, several studies utilizing only rigid (n = 6) cystoscopes [14,27,40,41,43] or only flexible (n = 3) cystoscopes [25,36,38] reported high therapeutic success and low adverse event rates.

Summary: The tolerability of a flexible vs. rigid cystoscopy during intravesical BTXA administration has not been directly studied, though both types are associated with good efficacy and low adverse rates.

3. Discussion

The variation in published BTXA injection techniques makes it difficult to effectively evaluate the impact of individual parameters. This challenge is further compounded by the heterogeneity of iOAB, which includes OAB-wet, characterized by UUI, and OAB-dry, defined by urgency and frequency without incontinence. Study outcomes also vary, with some focusing on UUI, urgency, or frequency and others on QOL parameters, making it difficult to compare efficacy and treatment outcomes across studies. These factors make it necessary to establish standardized injection protocols and consistent patient outcome reporting to allow for meaningful comparisons across studies.

Early dose-escalation studies established the dose–response relationship for reductions in UUI, leading to FDA approval of 100–200 U for iOAB due to its optimal balance of efficacy and safety [52]. While urinary retention, CIC, and UTI rates increase with higher doses, the benefits of dose escalation plateau above 200 U. In comparison to the 100 U dose, lower doses (50 U) reduce adverse events, but lack efficacy, whereas doses of 150 U provide marginal gains with a greater risk of complications. However, in select patients at higher risk of urinary retention, incremental dose adjustments may help optimize the balance between efficacy and adverse events. Dose selection should be individualized, considering patient-specific factors such as baseline post-void residual volume, risk of urinary retention, and tolerance for CIC. Further studies are needed to assess the role of lower doses (e.g., 50 U) in select patients at increased risk of urinary retention (e.g., males, frail, older adults, low Qmax and bladder contractility index [69], and to determine baseline factors (e.g., urodynamic parameters) that may predict success with the 50 U dose.

Similarly, trigone-sparing injections may offer potential benefits for iOAB patients at increased risk of retention. Studies comparing trigone-sparing and trigone-inclusive approaches suggest that including the trigone is safe and does not increase the risk of VUR. While trigone-including injections are effective, the addition of detrusor injections may increase the risk of voiding difficulty due to BTXA's impact on both motor and sensory neural pathways. In one study, the authors reported higher rates of subjective voiding difficulty and CIC with trigone-including detrusor injections compared to trigone-sparing detrusor injections [37]. However, CIC rates remained low (3.9%), and this difference was not observed in other studies included in our review. In contrast, trigone-inclusive bladder base injections without detrusor injections may result in lower rates of urinary retention requiring CIC compared to trigone-sparing detrusor injections, but they may be less durable [14,53]. This suggests that the trigone itself is not the critical factor, but rather that the distribution of motor neurons (e.g., detrusor vs. bladder base injections) is more important. Further adequately powered studies are needed to determine which iOAB patient populations would benefit most from detrusor, bladder base, or combination injection approaches.

Published studies use various combinations of injection depths, sites, numbers, and volumes, limiting our ability to draw clear conclusions on outcomes and adverse events. Individually, these variations do not appear to impact efficacy or adverse event rates. While the 20-injection regimen was most commonly used, alternative paradigms (1, 5, 10, 30, 40 injections) show similar efficacy and adverse events. One study (Liao 2016) found reduced efficacy with the 20-injection regimen compared to the 10- and 40-injection paradigms; however, the 20-injection group had less severe UUI at baseline [43]. In two mixed IDO and NDO cohort studies that did not meet the criteria for the current review, the authors found that fewer injections (1–4) had similar efficacy and duration of effect compared to 30 injection sites [70,71]. Overall, the literature on iOAB patients suggests that reducing the number of injections (1–10 injection) reduces procedure time, improving patient comfort and increasing willingness to repeat therapy [47,48]. Further adequately powered studies are needed to confirm these findings.

While the variations in injection numbers do not appear to impact efficacy or adverse event rates, further exploration into alternative injection approaches is warranted. One such approach, submucosal injections, may offer a promising alternative for tailored therapy in iOAB-dry patients by targeting sensory nerve activity while minimizing impact on detrusor contractility, as some residual BTXA likely diffuses across layers. A study by Kuo et al. suggests that suburothelial injections may be less durable than detrusor injections [53]. These findings suggest that injection depth may influence treatment efficacy, with detrusor injections showing greater durability compared to suburothelial injections. Adverse events, such as urinary retention, were more common in the detrusor and bladder body groups (13.3%, $n = 2/15$) than in the trigone-inclusive bladder base group (0%, $n = 0/15$), suggesting that the injection site may be more important than injection depth for urinary retention outcomes. In summary, injection depth (detrusor > suburothelial) appears to influence treatment durability, while injection site (bladder walls > base) appears more closely associated with urinary retention. However, this conclusion is based on two studies, and thus adequately powered studies are needed to clarify the impact of injection depth on both efficacy and urinary retention.

While injection depth and site may impact durability and retention rates, volume and distribution of injections (local vs. diffuse) are also critical for the spread of BTXA to presynaptic nerve terminals, located in the suburothelium and within the detrusor muscle. However, data on the impact of injection volume on efficacy and adverse events are limited due to the heterogeneity in injection site (e.g., trigone-only vs. non-trigone sparing approaches) and other interconnected parameters such as number of injections. The impact of volume on pain scores and tolerability remains underexplored in iOAB. Ton et al. evaluated 0.5 mL vs. 10 mL injection volumes, but did not assess pain or tolerability [48]. Similarly, there are limited data on how needle size affects BTXA outcomes or tolerability. The available literature suggests that ultrafine needles improve patient safety and comfort. A mixed IDO and NDO cohort study, which did not meet our scoping review inclusion criteria, utilized three needle sizes (22–27 gauge, 4–5 mm length) based on supply chain availability. VAS scores showed that the 27-gauge needle caused significantly less pain compared to larger needles [31]. Additionally, factors such as the number of injections (the first three were less painful than subsequent injections) and injection location (the posterior and right bladder wall were the most painful) also contributed to pain levels. One study investigated intravesical instillation of a BTXA + hydrogel admixture to see if injection can be avoided; however, there was no improvement over placebo [72]. No studies have directly compared BTXA tolerability, ease of administration, or efficacy between rigid and flexible scopes. While flexible scopes are assumed to be more comfortable [61,62], rigid scopes generally offer better control, are easier to use, and are generally lower in cost and maintenance.

Limitations of this scoping review include heterogeneity in BTXA injection paradigms, vague or inadequate reporting of study details, underpowered studies, heterogeneous patient populations (e.g., mixed cohorts of OAB-wet and OAB-dry), and non-standardized outcome measures. The variability in outcome definitions and measurement tools across included studies, particularly for QOL assessments, may affect the comparability of findings. However, this review offers potentially practice-altering insights, particularly regarding the impact of fewer injections and improved tolerability. Previously published recommendations for injection paradigms based on a combination of patient factors, available literature, and expert opinion may provide hypotheses to guide future studies (Table 2) [73]. The exclusion of non-English literature is also a limitation of this study, as it may have omitted relevant studies from the review.

Table 2. Proposed Botulinum Toxin Injection Paradigm Based on Patient Factors (Courtesy of Dr. Michael Kennelly, based on an assimilation of the literature and clinical practice on the use of BTXA over 20 years in the bladder for iOAB and Neurogenic Detrusor Overactivity).

	OAB Wet *	OAB Wet	OAB Wet	OAB Dry	NDO w CIC	NDO w/o CIC
BTX-A Naïve?	Yes	Yes	No	N/A	N/A	N/A
Dose (Units)	100	100	100–200	100	200–300	100
Location Detrusor vs. Submucosal	Detrusor	Detrusor	Detrusor	Submucosal	Submucosal	Submucosal
Trigone vs. Non-trigone	Both	Both	Both	Trigone	Non-trigone	Both
Distribution Local vs. Diffuse	Local	Diffuse	Diffuse	Local	Diffuse	Local
Number of injections	10	20	20	10	30	10
Dilution volume (mL)	0.5	0.5	1.0	0.5	1.0	1.0

* Patients at highest risk for incomplete bladder emptying (Diabetes Mellitus (DM), age > 70, Detrusor Hyperactivity with Impaired Contractile Function (DHIC), CIC averse).

4. Conclusions and Future Directions

Despite substantial evidence on dose–response relationships for UUI in managing refractory iOAB, significant gaps remain in individualizing therapy. Patient-specific factors, such as age, gender, comorbidities, urodynamic parameters, baseline bladder function, OAB subtype, and treatment history (e.g., BTXA-naïve patients), are insufficiently studied. Addressing these factors is essential for objectively assessing quality and outcomes in BTXA injection paradigms, ultimately informing clinical practice and patient counseling. The literature would benefit from future RCTs that assess the comparative impact of the number, volume, and site of Botox injections on treatment efficacy, tolerability, and the incidence of adverse events. Further research is needed to identify subgroups that may benefit from tailored doses, injection numbers, and scope types while balancing treatment effectiveness, adverse events, and tolerability. Establishing a standardized minimum dataset for this research (Table 3) would be beneficial. Similarly, future trials should focus on randomized controlled designs to assess individualized dosing strategies considering patient-specific factors. Exploring the economic impact of individualized therapy could yield healthcare savings, further supporting the optimization of treatment strategies. Additionally, establishing real-world data registries to track and evaluate long-term patient outcomes could provide valuable insights into the effectiveness and tolerability of botulinum toxin treatments across diverse populations.

Table 3. Proposed checklist for future Onabotulinum toxin A injection paradigm studies to ensure adequate reporting of study details.

Category	Details to Collect/Report
Methods	❑ Study Design (e.g., RCT, Prospective Cohort, Retrospective Cohort) ❑ Study Population ❑ Demographics (e.g., Age, Sex, Race/Ethnicity, Frailty status) ❑ OAB-wet vs. OAB-dry ❑ Other special populations ❑ Primary outcome ❑ Sample Size Calculation ❑ Follow up time
Procedure Details	❑ Anesthesia Details (choose 1 or more) ❑ Local anesthesia technique ❑ General Anesthesia ❑ Sedation details ❑ Dose (Units) ❑ Details of dilution strategy) (Units/mL) ❑ Anatomical location ❑ Trigone-inclusive ❑ Trigone sparing ❑ Number of injections ❑ Volume of injections ❑ Distribution of Injections ❑ Bladder base ❑ Bladder walls ❑ Both ❑ Spread of Injections ❑ Local ❑ Diffuse ❑ Procedure duration ❑ Needle gauge and length ❑ Scope type and sheath size

Table 3. *Cont.*

Category	Details to Collect/Report

Outcomes	Therapy Success
	❑ Subjective Outcomes
	  ❑ Validated questionnaires (PROs e.g., PGI-I, TBS, OAB-q, ICIQ-SF, OABSS, other relevant tools)
	❑ Objective Outcomes
	  ❑ Urgency, Urgency Incontinence, Micturition Episodes (e.g., Bladder diary)
	  ❑ UDS parameters
	❑ Other outcomes:
	  ❑ Pain/Tolerability (e.g., VAS, NPRS)
	  ❑ Willingness to repeat therapy
	  ❑ Time to next injection

Adverse Events	❑ Urinary retention requiring CIC ❑ UTI ❑ Hematuria

CIC: Clean Intermittent Catheterization, ICIQ-SF: International Consultation on Incontinence Questionnaire Short Form, NPRS: 11-point Numerical Pain Rating Scale, OABSS: Overactive Bladder Symptom Score, PGI-I: Patient Global Impression of Improvement, PROs: Patient Reported Outcomes, RCT: Randomized Controlled Trial, TBS: Treatment Benefit Scale, UDS: Urodynamic Study, UTI: Urinary Tract Infection. VAS: 10-point visual analog scale

5. Methodology

Given the heterogeneity of the available data, scoping review methodology was utilized. The standard methodology outlined in the Preferred Reporting Items for Systematic Reviews and Meta-Analyses (PRISMA) extension for Scoping Review checklist guidelines [74] was followed. The aim was to gain an overview of the current state of knowledge. We included studies that focused on idiopathic OAB patients receiving BTXA injection interventions without a comparison group, placebo, or alternative injection paradigm and reported efficacy and safety outcomes. This scoping review is not registered in PROSPERO, as scoping reviews are not currently accepted for registration under their criteria.

5.1. Study Selection

Inclusion Criteria: Our inclusion criteria were designed to encompass a broad range of studies relevant to the use of botulinum toxin, specifically BTXA, in treating idiopathic OAB in adult (>18 years) populations. We included studies involving idiopathic OAB and considered participants of both sexes without geographical restrictions. As this review was primarily focused on exploring the efficacy and safety of botulinum toxin, no specific comparison or control groups were mandated for inclusion. All papers published up until February 2024 were included (Table 1).

Exclusion Criteria: To ensure a comprehensive overview of the available literature, we considered all study designs except for systematic reviews, meta-analyses, scoping reviews, literature reviews, conference abstracts, case studies, and editorials. These criteria were established to prioritize primary research studies that provided substantive data relevant to the objectives of this review. Non-English language studies were excluded, as were those specifically addressing neurogenic detrusor overactivity. Furthermore, studies investigating botulinum toxin types other than BTXA were also excluded. Articles with no full-text accessibility were also excluded from the review.

5.2. Outcomes

The outcomes of interest included efficacy, including success rate, dry rate, and quality-of-life outcomes, and adverse events such as urinary tract infections, urinary retention, clean intermittent catheterization, and hematuria.

5.3. Search Strategy

Electronic databases, including PubMed, Embase, and Web of Science, were systematically searched by a trained librarian (AW) to identify relevant studies. Two reviewers manually removed 122 papers on neurogenic bladder during the full-text review.

A manual search of reference lists and relevant journals was conducted to supplement the electronic searches. Search terms were selected to encompass the breadth of relevant literature. They included phrases such as "overactive bladder", "idiopathic overactive bladder", "botulinum toxins", "Clostridium Botulinum", "Botulinum Neurotoxin", "Botox", and "OnabotulinumtoxinA". The Boolean operators AND, NOT, and OR were used to combine the search terms effectively.

5.4. Data Collection and Analysis

Four reviewers were engaged in the review process and independently assessed titles and abstracts using the Covidence platform. Full-text articles were then obtained and independently assessed for inclusion by two independent reviewers, and discrepancies were resolved through discussion with a third reviewer. Data extraction was conducted using Covidence to ensure systematic and organized collection of relevant information. A narrative synthesis approach was employed to summarize findings and identify key themes across the included studies.

Supplementary Materials: The following supporting information can be downloaded at https://www.mdpi.com/article/10.3390/toxins17050211/s1. Table S1: Data Extraction Table; Table S2: Injection Volume, Number, Depth and Location.

Author Contributions: Study design: E.E. and S.G. Collection and assembly of data: E.E., S.G. and H.M. Data analysis: E.E., S.G. and H.M. Data interpretation: E.E., S.G., H.M., S.S., V.H., R.S. and M.K. Manuscript preparation: E.E. and S.G. Manuscript review and revisions: E.E., S.G., H.M., S.S., V.H., R.S. and M.K. Final approval of manuscript: E.E., S.G., H.M., S.S., V.H., R.S. and M.K. All authors have read and agreed to the published version of the manuscript.

Funding: National Institutes of Health, National Institute of Diabetes and Digestive and Kidney Diseases, K23 DK131315.

Institutional Review Board Statement: Not applicable.

Informed Consent Statement: Not applicable.

Data Availability Statement: No new data were created or analyzed in this study.

Acknowledgments: We sincerely thank Amanda Woodward (AW) for assisting with the search strategy and literature search.

Conflicts of Interest: Ekene Enemchukwu: served on a research advisory board for Sumitomo pharma and Avation, received investigator-initiated research support from AbbVie and has received grant/research support from the National Institutes of Health. Michael Kennelly: advisory board and/or grant/research support from AbbVie, Axonics, Becton Dickinson, Coloplast, Cook Myosite, Medtronic, SpineX, and Urovant. The authors declare no conflict of interest.

References

1. Haylen, B.T.; de Ridder, D.; Freeman, R.M.; Swift, S.E.; Berghmans, B.; Lee, J.; Monga, A.; Petri, E.; Rizk, D.E.; Sand, P.K.; et al. An International Urogynecological Association (IUGA)/International Continence Society (ICS) joint report on the terminology for female pelvic floor dysfunction. *Int. Urogynecol. J.* **2010**, *21*, 5–26. [CrossRef] [PubMed]
2. Kocak, I.; Okyay, P.; Dundar, M.; Erol, H.; Beser, E. Female urinary incontinence in the west of Turkey: Prevalence, risk factors and impact on quality of life. *Eur. Urol.* **2005**, *48*, 634–641. [CrossRef]
3. Ninomiya, S.; Naito, K.; Nakanishi, K.; Okayama, H. Prevalence and Risk Factors of Urinary Incontinence and Overactive Bladder in Japanese Women. *Low. Urin. Tract. Symptoms* **2018**, *10*, 308–314. [CrossRef] [PubMed]
4. Chuang, Y.C.; Liu, S.P.; Lee, K.S.; Liao, L.; Wang, J.; Yoo, T.K.; Chu, R.; Sumarsono, B. Prevalence of overactive bladder in China, Taiwan and South Korea: Results from a cross-sectional, population-based study. *Low. Urin. Tract. Symptoms* **2019**, *11*, 48–55. [CrossRef] [PubMed]
5. Reynolds, W.S.; Fowke, J.; Dmochowski, R. The Burden of Overactive Bladder on US Public Health. *Curr. Bladder Dysfunct. Rep.* **2016**, *11*, 8–13. [CrossRef] [PubMed]
6. Stewart, W.F.; Van Rooyen, J.B.; Cundiff, G.W.; Abrams, P.; Herzog, A.R.; Corey, R.; Hunt, T.; Wein, A. Prevalence and burden of overactive bladder in the United States. *World J. Urol.* **2003**, *20*, 327–336. [CrossRef]
7. Coyne, K.S.; Sexton, C.C.; Vats, V.; Thompson, C.; Kopp, Z.S.; Milsom, I. National community prevalence of overactive bladder in the United States stratified by sex and age. *Urology* **2011**, *77*, 1081–1087. [CrossRef]
8. Chapple, C.; Sievert, K.D.; MacDiarmid, S.; Khullar, V.; Radziszewski, P.; Nardo, C.; Thompson, C.; Zhou, J.; Haag-Molkenteller, C. OnabotulinumtoxinA 100 U significantly improves all idiopathic overactive bladder symptoms and quality of life in patients with overactive bladder and urinary incontinence: A randomised, double-blind, placebo-controlled trial. *Eur. Urol.* **2013**, *6*[illegible], 249–256. [CrossRef]
9. Fowler, C.J.; Auerbach, S.; Ginsberg, D.; Hale, D.; Radziszewski, P.; Rechberger, T.; Patel, V.D.; Zhou, J.; Thompson, C.; Kowalski, J.W. OnabotulinumtoxinA improves health-related quality of life in patients with urinary incontinence due to idiopathic overactive bladder: A 36-week, double-blind, placebo-controlled, randomized, dose-ranging trial. *Eur. Urol.* **2012**, *62*, 148–157. [CrossRef]
10. Cameron, A.P.; Chung, D.E.; Dielubanza, E.J.; Enemchukwu, E.; Ginsberg, D.A.; Helfand, B.T.; Linder, B.J.; Reynolds, W.S.; Rovner, E.S.; Souter, L.; et al. The AUA/SUFU Guideline on the Diagnosis and Treatment of Idiopathic Overactive Bladder. *J Urol.* **2024**, *212*, 11–20. [CrossRef]
11. Nitti, V.W.; Dmochowski, R.; Herschorn, S.; Sand, P.; Thompson, C.; Nardo, C.; Yan, X.; Haag-Molkenteller, C.; EMBARK Study Group. OnabotulinumtoxinA for the treatment of patients with overactive bladder and urinary incontinence: Results of a phase 3, randomized, placebo controlled trial. *J. Urol.* **2013**, *189*, 2186–2193. [CrossRef] [PubMed]
12. McCammon, K.; Gousse, A.; Kohan, A.; Glazier, D.; Gruenenfelder, J.; Bai, Z.; Patel, A.M.; Hale, D. Early and Consistent Improvements in Urinary Symptoms and Quality of Life with OnabotulinumtoxinA in Patients with Overactive Bladder and Urinary Incontinence: Results from a Randomized, Placebo-controlled, Phase IV Clinical Trial. *Female Pelvic Med. Reconstr. Surg.* **2021**, *27*, 450–456. [CrossRef] [PubMed]
13. Bladder Wall—An Overview ScienceDirect Topics [Internet]. Available online: https://www.sciencedirect.com/topics/immunology-and-microbiology/bladder-wall (accessed on 10 March 2025).
14. Kuo, H.C. Comparison of effectiveness of detrusor, suburothelial and bladder base injections of botulinum toxin a for idiopathic detrusor overactivity. *J. Urol.* **2007**, *178 Pt 1*, 1359–1363. [CrossRef] [PubMed]
15. Karsenty, G.; Elzayat, E.; Delapparent, T.; St-Denis, B.; Lemieux, M.C.; Corcos, J. Botulinum toxin type a injections into the trigone to treat idiopathic overactive bladder do not induce vesicoureteral reflux. *J. Urol.* **2007**, *177*, 1011–1014. [CrossRef]
16. Coelho, A.; Dinis, P.; Pinto, R.; Gorgal, T.; Silva, C.; Silva, A.; Silva, J.; Cruz, C.D.; Cruz, F.; Avelino, A. Distribution of the high-affinity binding site and intracellular target of botulinum toxin type A in the human bladder. *Eur. Urol.* **2010**, *57*, 884–89[illegible]. [CrossRef]
17. Faure Walker, N.; Macpherson, F.; Tasleem, A.; Rampal, T. Interventions to improve tolerability of local anesthetic intradetrusor Botulinum toxin injections: A systematic review. *Neurourol. Urodyn.* **2023**, *42*, 23–32. [CrossRef]
18. Kelsey, E.; Wynn, J.; Holmes, A.; McLeod, K. Anatomical location and number of injection sites of intravesical OnabotulinumtoxinA for females with refractory idiopathic overactive bladder: A scoping review. *Neurourol. Urodyn.* **2024**, *43*, 553–5[illegible]. [CrossRef]
19. Karsenty, G.; Baverstock, R.; Carlson, K.; Diaz, D.C.; Cruz, F.; Dmochowski, R.; Fulford, S.; Giannantoni, A.; Heesakkers, J.; Kaufmann, A.; et al. Technical aspects of botulinum toxin type A injection in the bladder to treat urinary incontinence: Reviewing the procedure. *Int. J. Clin. Pract.* **2014**, *68*, 731–742. [CrossRef]
20. Jiang, Y.H.; Liao, C.H.; Kuo, H.C. Current and potential urological applications of botulinum toxin A. *Nat. Rev. Urol.* **2015**, *1*[illegible], 519–533. [CrossRef]
21. Jiang, Y.H.; Kuo, H.C. Reduction of urgency severity is the most important factor in the subjective therapeutic outcome of intravesical onabotulinumtoxinA injection for overactive bladder. *Neurourol Urodyn.* **2017**, *36*, 338–343. [CrossRef]

22. Hsiao, S.M.; Lin, H.H.; Kuo, H.C. Factors Associated with Therapeutic Efficacy of Intravesical OnabotulinumtoxinA Injection for Overactive Bladder Syndrome. *PLoS ONE* **2016**, *11*, e0147137. [CrossRef] [PubMed]
23. Available online: https://www.accessdata.fda.gov/drugsatfda_docs/label/2011/103000s5232lbl.pdf (accessed on 6 March 2025).
24. Rovner, E.; Kennelly, M.; Schulte-Baukloh, H.; Zhou, J.; Haag-Molkenteller, C.; Dasgupta, P. Urodynamic results and clinical outcomes with intradetrusor injections of onabotulinumtoxinA in a randomized, placebo-controlled dose-finding study in idiopathic overactive bladder. *Neurourol. Urodyn.* **2011**, *30*, 556–562. [CrossRef]
25. Ospina-Galeano, I.A.; Medina-Polo, J.; de la Rosa-Kerhmann, S.; Villacampa-Aubá, F.; Guerrero-Ramos, F.; Passas-Martínez, J.B. Use of onabotulinum toxin A in patients with idiopathic overactive bladder and a lack of efficacy, intolerance or contraindication with anticholinergics. *Rev. Urol. Colomb. Colomb. Urol. J.* **2018**, *27*, 86–91. [CrossRef]
26. Nitti, V.; Ginsberg, D.; Sievert, K.D.; Sussman, D.; Radomski, S.; Sand, P.; De Ridder, D.; Jenkins, B.; Magyar, A.; Chapple, C. Durable Efficacy and Safety of Long-Term OnabotulinumtoxinA Treatment in Patients with Overactive Bladder Syndrome: Final Results of a 3.5-Year Study. *J. Urol.* **2016**, *196*, 791–800. [CrossRef]
27. Karakeçi, A.; Keleş, A.; Ozan, T.; Firdolaş, F.; Onur, R. Efficacy and Safety of Botulinum Neurotoxin in Geriatric Patients with an Overactive Bladder: A Multicentric Study from Turkey. *Turk. J. Geriatr.* **2019**, *22*, 197–204. [CrossRef]
28. Yokoyama, O.; Honda, M.; Yamanishi, T.; Sekiguchi, Y.; Fujii, K.; Nakayama, T.; Mogi, T.; Kitta, T.; Ohyama, C.; Kambe, K.; et al. OnabotulinumtoxinA (botulinum toxin type A) for the treatment of Japanese patients with overactive bladder and urinary incontinence: Results of single-dose treatment from a phase III, randomized, double-blind, placebo-controlled trial (interim analysis). *Int. J. Urol. Off. J. Jpn. Urol. Assoc.* **2020**, *27*, 227–234. [CrossRef] [PubMed]
29. Singh, R.; El Nashar, S.A.; Trabuco, E.C.; Klingele, C.J.; Gebhart, J.B.; Occhino, J.A. Comparison of Short Term Outcomes of Sacral Nerve Stimulation and Intradetrusor Injection of OnabotulinumtoxinA (Botox) in Women With Refractory Overactive Bladder. *Female Pelvic Med. Reconstr. Surg.* **2015**, *21*, 369–373. [CrossRef]
30. Sievert, K.D.; Chapple, C.; Herschorn, S.; Joshi, M.; Zhou, J.; Nardo, C.; Nitti, V.W. OnabotulinumtoxinA 100U provides significant improvements in overactive bladder symptoms in patients with urinary incontinence regardless of the number of anticholinergic therapies used or reason for inadequate management of overactive bladder. *Int. J. Clin. Pract.* **2014**, *68*, 1246–1256. [CrossRef]
31. Schulte-Baukloh, H.; Weiß, C.; Weinberger, S.; Hubatsch, M.; Schlomm, T.; Ralla, B. Real-Time Documentation of the Effect of Onabotulinumtoxin A Detrusor Injection in OAB Patients—Preliminary Results. *Toxins* **2022**, *15*, 30. [CrossRef]
32. Onem, K.; Bayrak, O.; Demirtas, A.; Coskun, B.; Dincer, M.; Kocak, I.; Onur, R. Efficacy and safety of onabotulinumtoxinA injection in patients with refractory overactive bladder: First multicentric study in Turkish population. *Neurourol. Urodyn.* **2018**, *37*, 263–268. [CrossRef]
33. Okamura, K.; Takei, M.; Nojiri, Y.; Otsuka, A.; Takamoto, H.; Maeda, Y.; Fujimura, T.; Yokoyama, T.; Gotoh, M.; Homma, Y. Twelve Months Follow-up of Injection of OnabotulinumtoxinA into Vesical Submucosa for Refractory Non-neurogenic Overactive Bladder. *Low. Urin. Tract. Symptoms* **2013**, *5*, 55–59. [CrossRef] [PubMed]
34. Mühlstädt, S.; Mischner, S.; Kranz, J.; Anheuser, P.; Mohammed, N.; Steffens, J.A.; Fornara, P. Quo Vadis Botulinum Toxin: Normative Constraints and Quality of Life for Patients with Idiopathic OAB? *Front. Surg.* **2018**, *5*, 61. [CrossRef]
35. MacDiarmid, S.; Glazier, D.B.; McCrery, R.J.; Kennelly, M.J.; Nelson, M.; Ifantides, K.B.; McCammon, K.A. Efficacy and safety of an alternative onabotulinumtoxinA injection paradigm for refractory overactive bladder. *Neurourol. Urodyn.* **2024**, *43*, 31–43. [CrossRef]
36. Granese, R.; Adile, G.; Gugliotta, G.; Cucinella, G.; Saitta, S.; Adile, B. Botox(®) for idiopathic overactive bladder: Efficacy, duration and safety. Effectiveness of subsequent injection. *Arch. Gynecol. Obstet.* **2012**, *286*, 923–929. [CrossRef]
37. El-Hefnawy, A.S.; Elbaset, M.A.; Taha, D.E.; Wadie, B.S.; Kenawy, M.; Shokeir, A.A.; Badry, M.E. Trigonal-sparing versus trigonal-involved Botox injection for treatment of idiopathic overactive bladder: A randomized clinical trial. *Low. Urin. Tract. Symptoms* **2021**, *13*, 22–30. [CrossRef]
38. Cohen, B.L.; Barboglio, P.; Rodriguez, D.; Gousse, A.E. Preliminary results of a dose-finding study for botulinum toxin-A in patients with idiopathic overactive bladder: 100 versus 150 units. *Neurourol. Urodyn.* **2009**, *28*, 205–208. [CrossRef]
39. AlTaweel, W.; Mokhtar, A.; Rabah, D.M. Prospective randomized trial of 100u vs. 200u botox in the treatment of idiopathic overactive bladder. *Urol. Ann.* **2011**, *3*, 66. [CrossRef]
40. Abdelwahab, O.; Sherif, H.; Soliman, T.; Elbarky, I.; Eshazly, A. Efficacy of botulinum toxin type A 100 Units versus 200 units for treatment of refractory idiopathic overactive bladder. *Int. Braz. J. Urol. Off. J. Braz. Soc. Urol.* **2015**, *41*, 1132–1140. [CrossRef]
41. Ou, Y.C.; Kao, Y.L.; Ho, Y.H.; Wu, K.Y.; Kuo, H.C. Intravesical Injection of Botulinum Toxin Type A in Patients with Refractory Overactive Bladder-Results between Young and Elderly Populations, and Factors Associated with Unfavorable Outcomes. *Toxins* **2023**, *15*, 95. [CrossRef] [PubMed]
42. DiCarlo-Meacham, A.M.; Dengler, K.L.; Welch, E.K.; Brooks, D.I.; Gruber, D.D.; Osborn, D.J.; Scarlotta, L.; Vaccaro, C.M. Reduced versus standard intradetrusor OnabotulinumtoxinA injections for treatment of overactive bladder. *Neurourol. Urodyn.* **2023**, *42*, 366–374. [CrossRef] [PubMed]

43. Liao, C.H.; Chen, S.F.; Kuo, H.C. Different number of intravesical onabotulinumtoxinA injections for patients with refractory detrusor overactivity do not affect treatment outcome: A prospective randomized comparative study. *Neurourol. Urodyn.* **2016**, *35*, 717–723. [CrossRef]
44. Owen, R.K.; Abrams, K.R.; Mayne, C.; Slack, M.; Tincello, D.G. Comparison of the effectiveness of repeated injections of onabotulinum toxin A for refractory idiopathic detrusor overactivity: Analysis of an open label extension of a randomized trial (the RELAX study). *Neurourol. Urodyn.* **2017**, *36*, 1201–1207. [CrossRef]
45. Mohanty, N.K.; Nayak, R.L.; Alam, M.; Arora, R.P. Role of botulinum toxin-A in management of refractory idiopathic detrusor overactive bladder: Single center experience. *Indian J. Urol. J. Urol. Soc. India* **2008**, *24*, 182–185. [CrossRef] [PubMed]
46. Kuschel, S.; Werner, M.; Schmid, D.M.; Faust, E.; Schuessler, B. Botulinum toxin-A for idiopathic overactivity of the vesical detrusor: A 2-year follow-up. *Int. Urogynecol. J. Pelvic. Floor Dysfunct.* **2008**, *19*, 905–909. [CrossRef]
47. Chang, E.S.; Ringel, N.; Woodburn, K.L.; Tanner, J.P.; Bassaly, R.; Greene, K.; Wyman, A.; Iglesia, C. Postprocedural Pain Associated with 5 Versus 20 Intradetrusor Injections of onabotulinumtoxinA for Treatment of Overactive Bladder: A Multicenter Randomized Clinical Trial. *Urogynecology* **2022**, *28*, 518–525. [CrossRef] [PubMed]
48. Ton, J.; Downing, P.; Versi, E.; van Uem, S.; Ephraim, S.; Murphy, M.; Lucente, V. Outcomes of a single trigone-only vs. 20 trigone-sparing injections of OnabotulinumtoxinA for refractory overactive bladder (OAB). *Int. Urol. Nephrol.* **2021**, *53*, 1067–1072. [CrossRef]
49. Zdroik, A.; El Haraki, A.; Smith, W.; Badlani, G.; Parker-Autry, C.; Matthews, C. Injection site number and outcomes of intradetrusor onabotulinumtoxinA for refractory overactive bladder syndrome: A randomized clinical trial. *Int. Urogynecol. J.* **2024**, *35*, 119–126. [CrossRef]
50. Herschorn, S.; Kohan, A.; Aliotta, P.; McCammon, K.; Sriram, R.; Abrams, S.; Lam, W.; Everaert, K. The Efficacy and Safety of OnabotulinumtoxinA or Solifenacin Compared with Placebo in Solifenacin Naïve Patients with Refractory Overactive Bladder: Results from a Multicenter, Randomized, Double-Blind Phase 3b Trial. *J. Urol.* **2017**, *198*, 167–175. [CrossRef]
51. Tamburro, F.R.; Castellan, P.; Neri, F.; Berardinelli, F.; Bada, M.; Sountoulides, P.; Giuliani, N.; Agrò, E.F.; Schips, L.; Cindolo, L. Onabotulinumtoxin-A improves health status and urinary symptoms in subjects with refractory overactive bladder: Real-life experience. *Urol. J.* **2018**, *85*, 163–168. [CrossRef] [PubMed]
52. Dmochowski, R.; Chapple, C.; Nitti, V.W.; Chancellor, M.; Everaert, K.; Thompson, C.; Daniell, G.; Zhou, J.; Haag-Molkenteller, C. Efficacy and safety of onabotulinumtoxinA for idiopathic overactive bladder: A double-blind, placebo controlled, randomized, dose ranging trial. *J. Urol.* **2010**, *184*, 2416–2422. [CrossRef]
53. Kuo, H.C. Bladder base/trigone injection is safe and as effective as bladder body injection of onabotulinumtoxinA for idiopathic detrusor overactivity refractory to antimuscarinics. *Neurourol. Urodyn.* **2011**, *30*, 1242–1248. [CrossRef]
54. Ginsberg, D.A.; Drake, M.J.; Kaufmann, A.; Radomski, S.; Gousse, A.E.; Chermansky, C.J.; Magyar, A.; Nicandro, J.P.; Nitti, V.W. 191622-096 Investigators. Long-Term Treatment with OnabotulinumtoxinA Results in Consistent, Durable Improvements in Health Related Quality of Life in Patients with Overactive Bladder. *J. Urol.* **2017**, *198*, 897–904. [CrossRef] [PubMed]
55. El-Azab, A.S.; Moeen, A.M. The satisfaction of patients with refractory idiopathic overactive bladder with onabotulinumtoxinA and augmentation cystoplasty. *Arab. J. Urol.* **2013**, *11*, 344–349. [CrossRef] [PubMed]
56. Flynn, M.K.; Amundsen, C.L.; Perevich, M.; Liu, F.; Webster, G.D. Outcome of a randomized, double-blind, placebo controlled trial of botulinum A toxin for refractory overactive bladder. *J. Urol.* **2009**, *181*, 2608–2615. [CrossRef] [PubMed]
57. Amundsen, C.L.; Richter, H.E.; Menefee, S.A.; Komesu, Y.M.; Arya, L.A.; Gregory, W.T.; Myers, D.L.; Zyczynski, H.M.; Vasavada, S.; Nolen, T.L.; et al. OnabotulinumtoxinA vs. Sacral Neuromodulation on Refractory Urgency Urinary Incontinence in Women: A Randomized Clinical Trial. *JAMA* **2016**, *316*, 1366–1374. [CrossRef]
58. Brubaker, L.; Richter, H.E.; Visco, A.; Mahajan, S.; Nygaard, I.; Braun, T.M.; Barber, M.D.; Menefee, S.; Schaffer, J.; Weber, A.M.; et al. Refractory idiopathic urge urinary incontinence and botulinum A injection. *J. Urol.* **2008**, *180*, 217–222. [CrossRef]
59. Apostolidis, A.; Dasgupta, P.; Denys, P.; Elneil, S.; Fowler, C.J.; Giannantoni, A.; Karsenty, G.; Schulte-Baukloh, H.; Schurch, B.; Wyndaele, J.J. Recommendations on the use of botulinum toxin in the treatment of lower urinary tract disorders and pelvic floor dysfunctions: A European consensus report. *Eur. Urol.* **2009**, *55*, 100–119. [CrossRef]
60. Dasgupta, P. Volume matters: Bladder injections of botulinum toxin type A. *Eur. Urol.* **2012**, *61*, 1185–1186; discussion 1886–1887. [CrossRef]
61. Denholm, S.W.; Conn, I.G.; Newsam, J.E.; Chisholm, G.D. Morbidity following cystoscopy: Comparison of flexible and rigid techniques. *Br. J. Urol.* **1990**, *66*, 152–154. [CrossRef]
62. Flannigan, G.M.; Gelister, J.S.; Noble, J.G.; Milroy, E.J. Rigid versus flexible cystoscopy. A controlled trial of patient tolerance. *Br. J. Urol.* **1988**, *62*, 537–540. [CrossRef]
63. Krajewski, W.; Zdrojowy, R.; Wojciechowska, J.; Kościelska, K.; Dembowski, J.; Matuszewski, M.; Tupikowski, K.; Małkiewicz, B.; Kołodziej, A. Patient comfort during flexible and rigid cystourethroscopy. *Wideochirurgia Inne Tech. Maloinwazyjne Videosurgery Miniinvasive Tech.* **2016**, *11*, 94–97. [CrossRef]

64. Seklehner, S.; Remzi, M.; Fajkovic, H.; Saratlija-Novakovic, Z.; Skopek, M.; Resch, I.; Duvnjak, M.; Hruby, S.; Librenjak, D.; Hübner, W.; et al. Prospective multi-institutional study analyzing pain perception of flexible and rigid cystoscopy in men. *Urology* **2015**, *85*, 737–741. [CrossRef] [PubMed]
65. Casteleijn, N.F.; Vriesema, J.L.; Stomps, S.P.; van Balen, O.L.W.B.; Cornel, E.B. The effect of office based flexible and rigid cystoscopy on pain experience in female patients. *Investig. Clin. Urol.* **2017**, *58*, 48–53. [CrossRef]
66. Feng, D.; Chen, G.; Yang, Y.; Wei, W.; Wei, X. Does office-based flexible cystoscopy provide better pain perception than rigid cystoscopy: A systematic review and meta-analysis. *Ann. Palliat. Med.* **2021**, *10*, 6228–6235. [CrossRef] [PubMed]
67. Ucer, O.; Temeltas, G.; Gumus, B.; Muezzinoglu, T. Comparison of pain, quality of life, lower urinary tract symptoms and sexual function between flexible and rigid cystoscopy in follow-up male patients with non muscle invasive bladder cancer: A randomized controlled cross section single blind study. *Int. J. Clin. Pract.* **2021**, *75*, e13853. [CrossRef] [PubMed]
68. Gee, J.R.; Waterman, B.J.; Jarrard, D.F.; Hedican, S.P.; Bruskewitz, R.C.; Nakada, S.Y. Flexible and rigid cystoscopy in women. *J. Soc. Laparoendosc. Surg.* **2009**, *13*, 135–138.
69. Abrar, M.; Pindoria, N.; Malde, S.; Chancellor, M.; DeRidder, D.; Sahai, A. Predictors of Poor Response and Adverse Events Following Botulinum Toxin A for Refractory Idiopathic Overactive Bladder: A Systematic Review. *Eur. Urol. Focus* **2021**, *7*, 1448–1467. [CrossRef]
70. Martínez-Cuenca, E.; Bonillo, M.A.; Morán, E.; Broseta, E.; Arlandis, S. Onabotulinumtoxina Re-Injection for Refractory Detrusor Overactivity Using 3-4 Injection Sites: Results of a Pilot Study. *Urology* **2020**, *137*, 50–54. [CrossRef]
71. Avallone, M.A.; Sack, B.S.; El-Arabi, A.; Guralnick, M.L.; O'Connor, R.C. Less is more-A pilot study evaluating one to three intradetrusor sites for injection of OnabotulinumtoxinA for neurogenic and idiopathic detrusor overactivity. *Neurourol. Urodyn.* **2017**, *36*, 1104–1107. [CrossRef]
72. Chermansky, C.J.; Richter, H.E.; Jacoby, K.; Titanji, W.; Jenkins, B.; Geib, T.; Brucker, B.M. Intravesical Instillation of OnabotulinumtoxinA in the Treatment of Refractory Overactive Bladder in Participants with Urinary Incontinence. *J. Urol.* **2022**, *208*, 855–862. [CrossRef]
73. Impact of Technique on Outcomes of Botulinum Toxin Injection for Idiopathic Overactive Bladder—American Urological Association [Internet]. [Cited 6 March 2025]. Available online: https://auanews.net/issues/articles/2022/february-2022/impact-of-technique-on-outcomes-of-botulinum-toxin-injection-for-idiopathic-overactive-bladder (accessed on 6 March 2025).
74. Tricco, A.C.; Lillie, E.; Zarin, W.; O'Brien, K.K.; Colquhoun, H.; Levac, D.; Moher, D.; Peters, M.D.; Horsley, T.; Weeks, L.; et al. PRISMA Extension for Scoping Reviews (PRISMA-ScR): Checklist and Explanation. *Ann. Intern. Med.* **2018**, *169*, 467–473. [CrossRef] [PubMed]

MDPI AG
Grosspeteranlage 5
4052 Basel
Switzerland
Tel.: +41 61 683 77 34

Toxins Editorial Office
E-mail: toxins@mdpi.com
www.mdpi.com/journal/toxins

www.ingramcontent.com/pod-product-compliance
Lightning Source LLC
Chambersburg PA
CBHW062057220926
51850CB00010B/2797
* 9 7 8 3 7 2 5 8 6 3 3 8 9 *